Chronic Obstructive Pulmonary Disease - A Current Conspectus

Edited by Kian Chung Ong

Published in London, United Kingdom

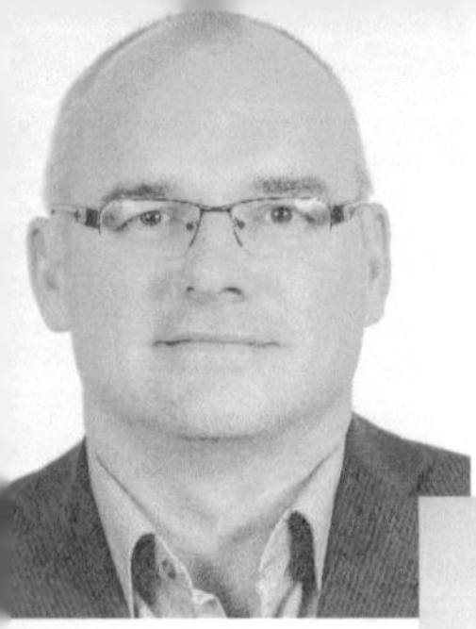
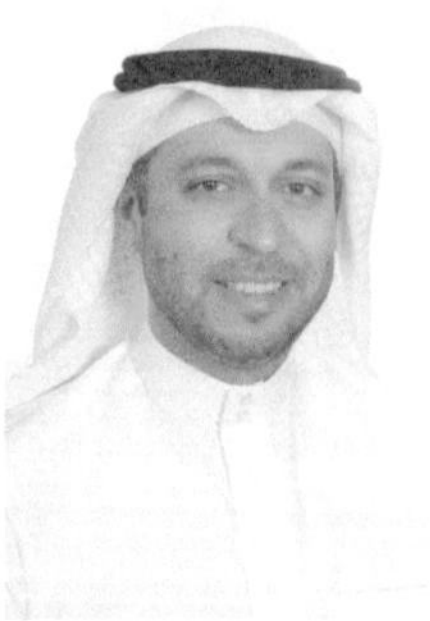
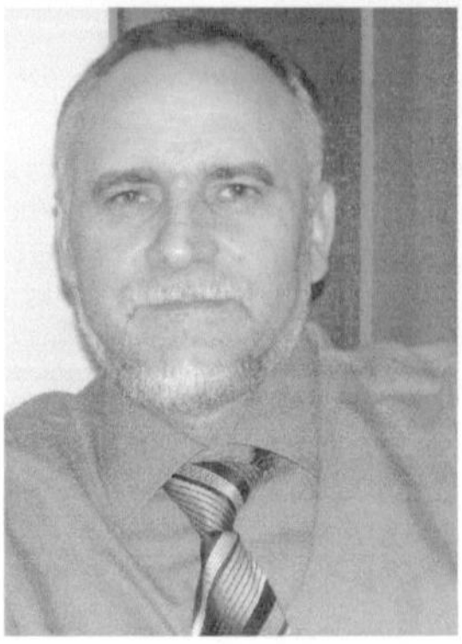
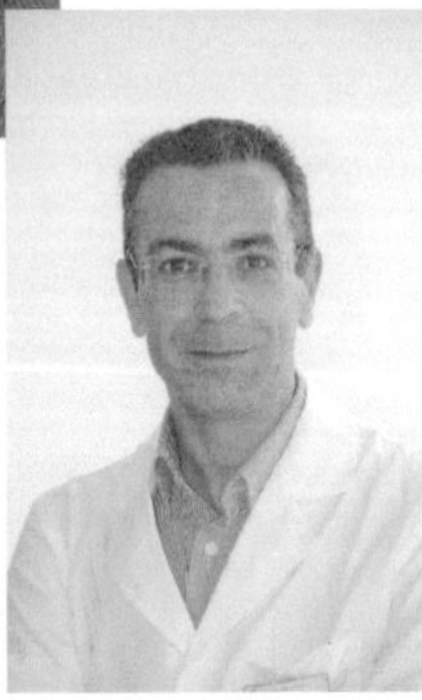
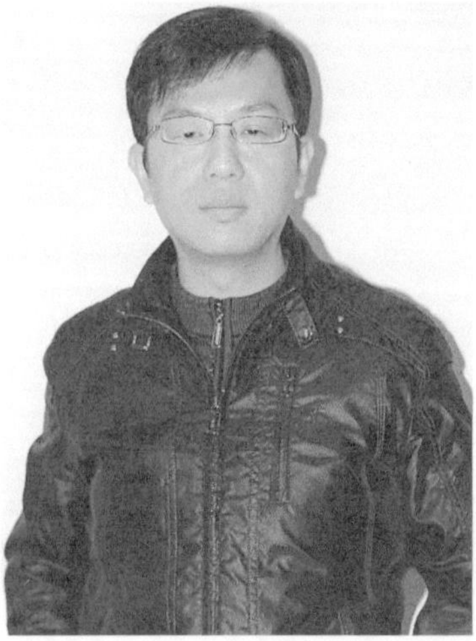
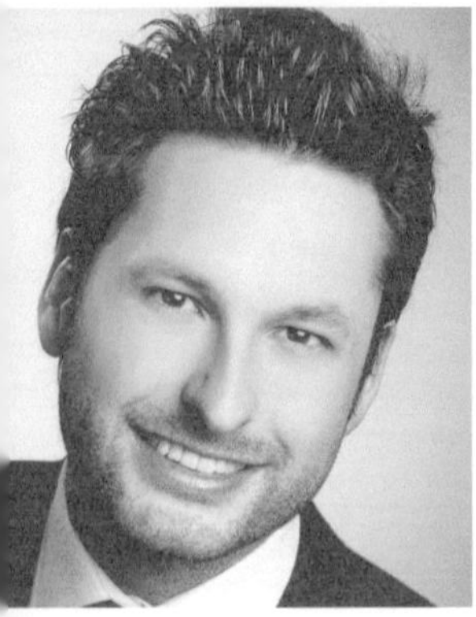
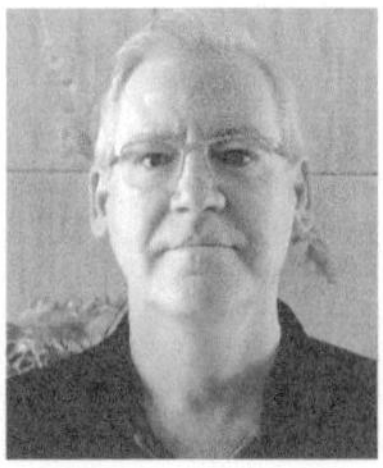

IntechOpen

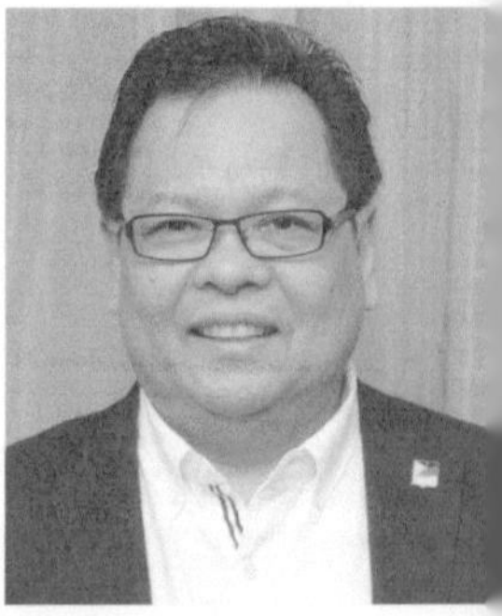
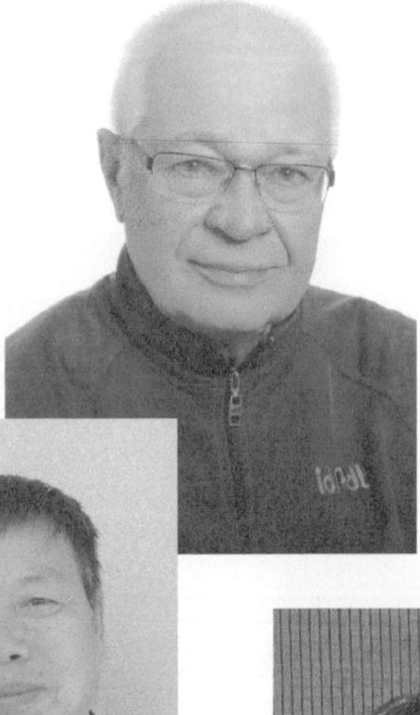
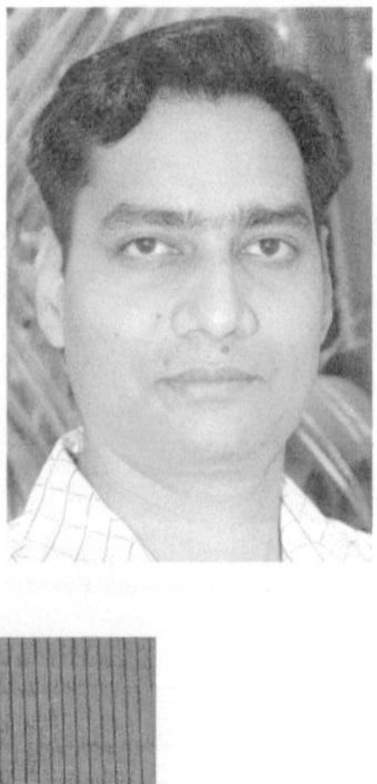
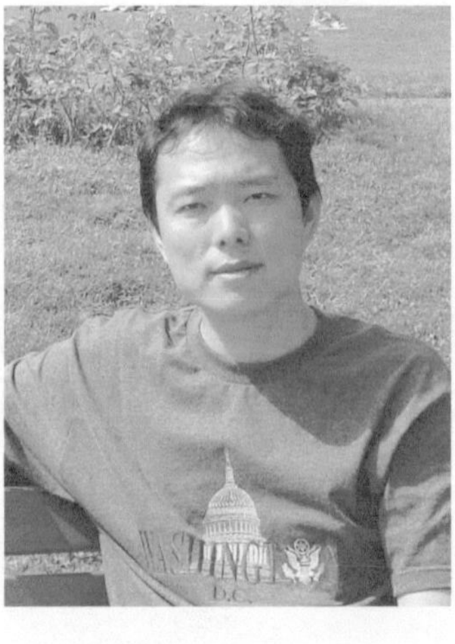
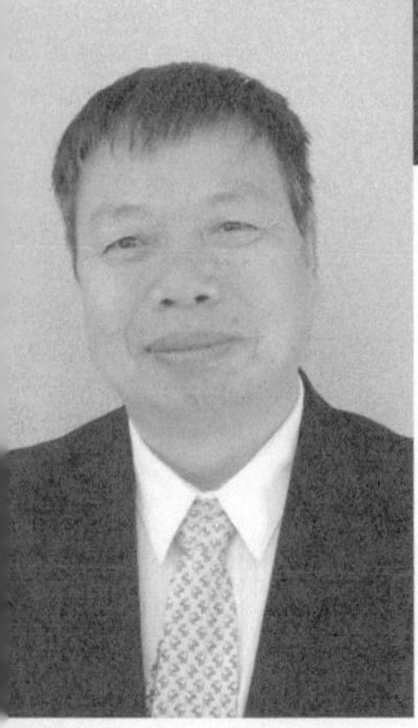
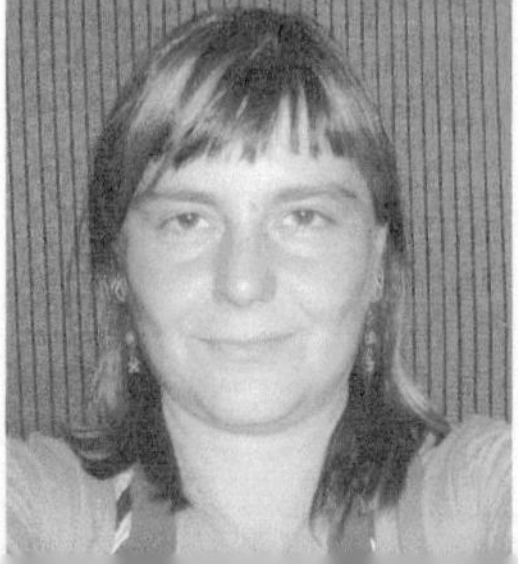

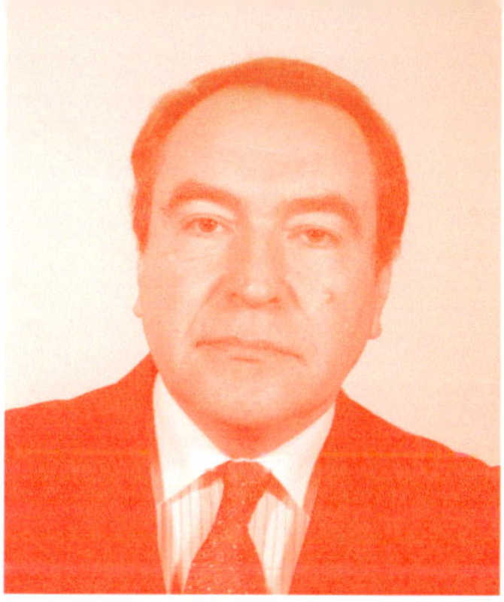

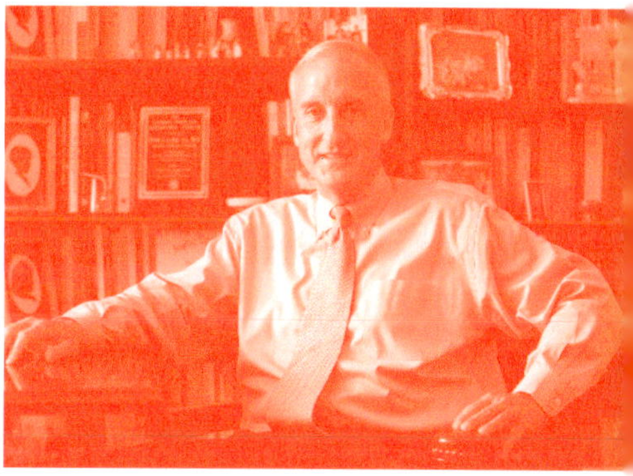

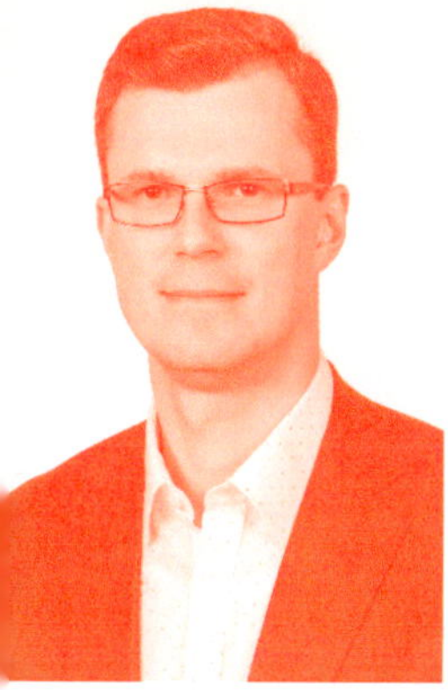

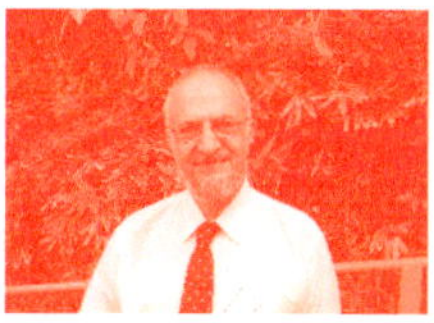

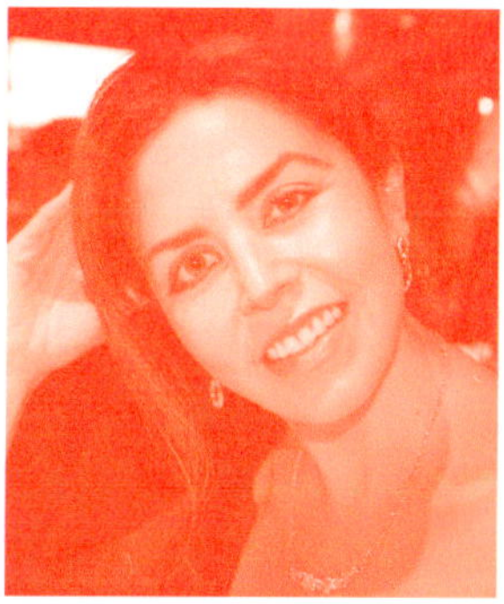

Supporting open minds since 2005

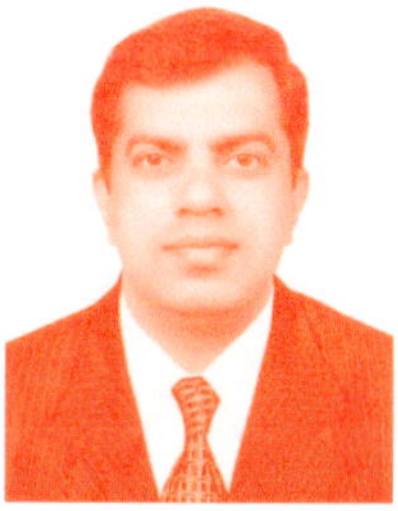

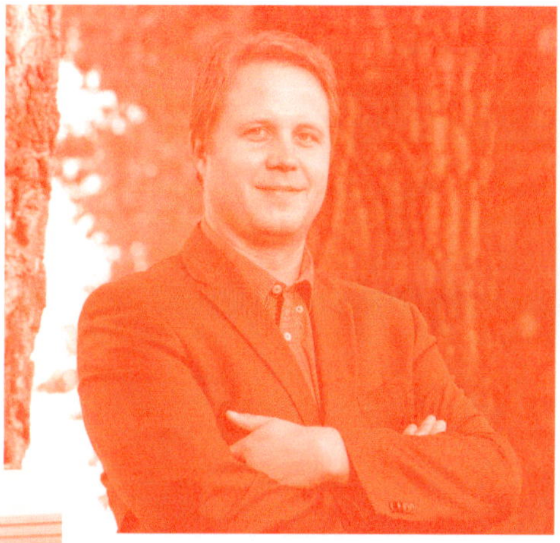

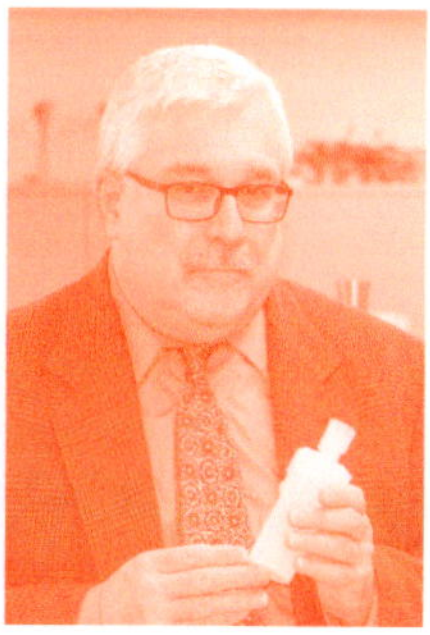

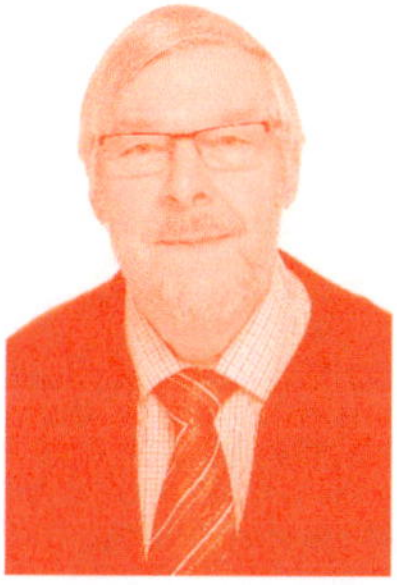

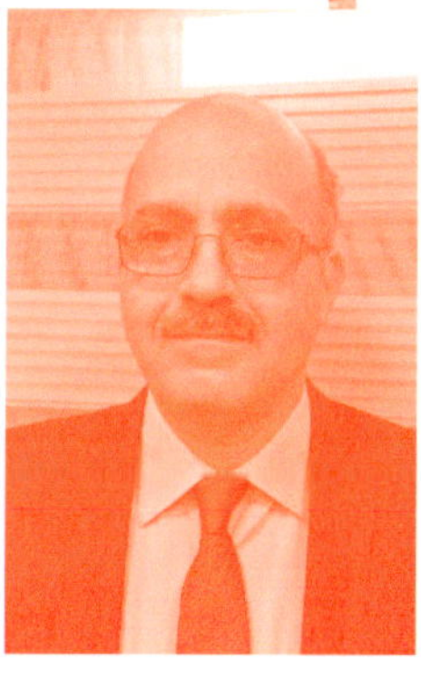

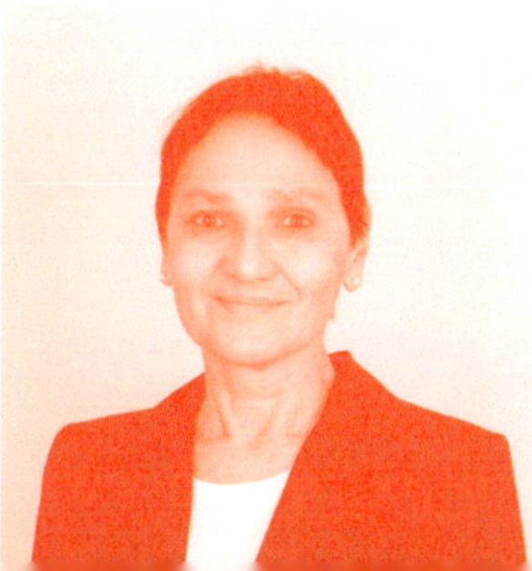

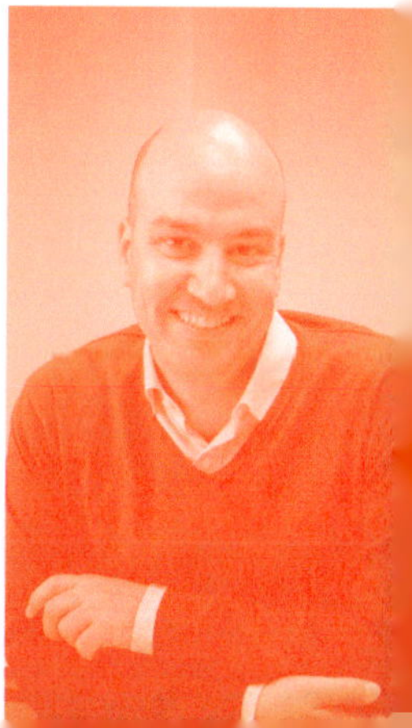

Chronic Obstructive Pulmonary Disease - A Current Conspectus
http://dx.doi.org/10.5772/intechopen.91516
Edited by Kian Chung Ong

Contributors
Anca Mihaela Hâncu, Florin Dumitru Mihălţan, Maria Mota, Mihaela Vladu, Özlem Ediboğlu, Carlos A. Torres-Duque, Felipe Severiche-Bueno, Mauricio Gonzalez-Garcia, Amira Permatasari Tarigan, Fannie Rizki Ananda, Annie Heiderscheit, Biruk Getahun, Abebe Ayalew Bekel, Maha Dardouri, Manel Mallouli, Kian Chung Ong

First published in London, United Kingdom, 2021 by IntechOpen
IntechOpen is the global imprint of INTECHOPEN LIMITED, registered in England and Wales, registration number: 11086078, 5 Princes Gate Court, London, SW7 2QJ, United Kingdom
Printed in Croatia

British Library Cataloguing-in-Publication Data
A catalogue record for this book is available from the British Library

Additional hard and PDF copies can be obtained from orders@intechopen.com

Chronic Obstructive Pulmonary Disease - A Current Conspectus
Edited by Kian Chung Ong
p. cm.
Print ISBN 978-1-83968-926-0
Online ISBN 978-1-83968-927-7
eBook (PDF) ISBN 978-1-83968-928-4

For EU product safety concerns:
IN TECH d.o.o., Prolaz Marije Krucifikse Kozulić 3, 51000 Rijeka, Croatia, info@intechopen.com or visit our website at intechopen.com.

Meet the editor

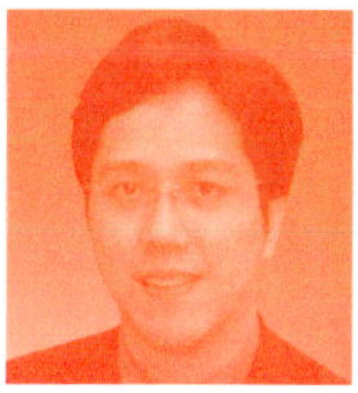

Dr. Ong is a respiratory physician and intensivist with more than twenty years of experience. He is currently the medical director of Chestmed Pte Ltd, Mount Elizabeth Medical Centre, Singapore. He is also the founding and current president of the Chronic Obstructive Pulmonary Disease Association (Singapore) and is a member of the Global Initiative for Chronic Obstructive Lung Disease (GOLD) Assembly. He is the principal author of multiple publications in international peer-reviewed medical journals such as *CHEST*, *European Respiratory Journal*, *American Journal of Respiratory and Critical Care Medicine*, and *Respiratory Medicine*. He is also the editor of the textbook *Chronic Obstructive Pulmonary Disease – Current Concepts and Practice*.

Contents

Preface

This book was produced during a challenging time. One and a half years into a pandemic that has taken the world by surprise, the medical community continues to cope with the travails caused by the novel severe acute respiratory syndrome coronavirus 2 (SARS-CoV-2). As countries around the world concentrate their resources to battle this pandemic, there will almost inevitably be collateral damage brought about by friendly fire. Funding for and research in other medical conditions are put aside, as priorities in healthcare expenditure are re-arranged. One such major medical condition likely to incur indirect losses during the current pandemic is Chronic Obstructive Pulmonary Disease (COPD). At the time of this writing, COPD remains the third leading cause of death worldwide and continues to claim more lives than all respiratory tract infections (inclusive of deaths due to the viral pandemic). COPD has been deprived of apposite attention despite its major contribution to the global disease burden and is likely to accede to further diversion of attention and resources due to the current pandemic. In such trying times, I humbly acknowledge the significance of disseminating erudite information on COPD via an open-access manner.

COPD is a disease that is multi-factorial in etiology, effects multi-systemic involvement, and requires multi-modality management. It is difficult to find another respiratory disorder that affects so many individuals in such a multi-dimensional way. In managing COPD, healthcare professionals hail from diverse backgrounds ranging from smoking cessation therapists to statisticians, pharmacists to physiotherapists, respiratory physicians to rehabilitation specialists, investigators to intensivists, and more. Over time, such diversity in unity has led to the development of a widespread community involved in the treatment of COPD. Members of this community from all around the world had contributed to an earlier book by the same publisher titled *Chronic Obstructive Pulmonary Disease – Current Concepts and Practice*, a book that has been well received, judging from the number of copies that have been downloaded and read thus far. This current conspectus is an up-to-date codicil to the former book and the present iteration has received contributions from the eclectic community involved in the management of COPD.

The introductory chapter emphasizes the importance of a global and multi-dimensional enterprise in confronting COPD, together with merging the old (experience) with the new (technology). Chapters 2 and 3 examine the multi-factorial causes leading to the development of COPD. In Chapter 2, the authors emphasize that exposure to tobacco smoke is not necessarily the *sine qua non* of COPD and the disease should not be depicted as self-inflicted, as factors such as air pollution and work-related exposures are major causes of COPD in many parts of the world. The authors compare and contrast heterogeneity of COPD caused by smoke from cigarettes and biomass fuel according to pathogenesis and presentation. The impact of occupational exposures in disease burden and work performance is exposited in Chapter 3. Chapter 4 examines disease-related contributors to health status in COPD with the aim of discovering elements that impact patients' lives the most. Chapter 5 discusses the holistic management of COPD patients including exercise training in the context of pulmonary rehabilitation targeted at improving lung function. Chapter 6 discusses nutritional interventions and weight management. Chapter 7 examines the complexities of mechanical ventilation in COPD, and finally, Chapter 8 discusses the plausibility of reducing stress and improving outcomes in COPD patients on mechanical ventilation by the innovative use of patient-directed music listening.

In addition to the invaluable contributions of the chapter authors, I am indebted to Ms. Maja Bozicevic and her team of editorial assistants at IntechOpen, without whom this book would not have been produced expediently in such challenging circumstances.

Kian-Chung Ong
Mount Elizabeth Medical Centre,
Singapore

Chapter 1

Introductory Chapter: Confronting COPD by Merging Experience with Enterprise

Kian-Chung Ong

1. Introduction

1.1 Combining experience and enterprise

The general backdrop in the management of Chronic Obstructive Pulmonary Disease (COPD) has remarkably transformed in the past two decades. Gone is the erstwhile nihilistic outlook of COPD as this is replaced by fresh optimism in the approach to curtailing the disease [1]. Among the newer developments in recent years that led to increased alacrity in confronting a disease that continues to defy efforts aimed at reducing its morbidity and mortality is the recognition that people all around the globe can play significant roles in reducing the COPD disease burden [2]. Leading the charge in this global enterprise are, quite expectedly, the front-line healthcare professionals who are bearing the load of caring for multitudes of patients suffering from the disease. Undaunted by the inundation of challenges posed by this disease, clinicians have been energized to assume additional roles over and above their duty of care. Many experienced and leading clinicians have gathered together multi-disciplinary local and international organizations that contribute to the advocacy, research, education, and development of clinical practice guidelines on COPD. The recent trend of identifying and managing "treatable traits" in respiratory disease is a prime example of initiatives started by experienced pulmonologists that led to major cooperation and knowledge transfer, resulting in major paradigm shifts in the management of COPD. Identifying a simple biomarker like peripheral eosinophilia that is related to important clinical events such as exacerbation rates and is responsive to treatment with steroids has had major impact on symptoms and progression of the disease.

Another potential contribution from experienced clinicians in the field of respiratory medicine is in the exponential development of digital technologies in Respiratory Medicine. For the novice in medical technology, the following are broad categories of digital development in the field of respiratory medicine:

1. Telemedicine – this includes tele-consultation, tele-monitoring and tele-rehabilitation, all increasing in demand with the current pandemic

2. Artificial Intelligence (AI) – current uses include Google AI that has been shown to be as good as or better in diagnosing/predicting lung cancer using screening CT scans than traditional reporting by radiologists. Google Augmented Reality (AR) microscope also are less likely to miss cancer diagnosis, reducing the workload of pathologists

IntechOpen

3. Digital diagnosis – software systems that provide diagnosis of medical conditions using available information without human doctors

4. Equipment software – mobile health or m-health, the practice of medicine or public health supported by mobile devices

5. Medical robotics – including use of virtual reality & mixed reality that allows interaction with the user (e.g. surgeons during procedures)

6. Others e.g. Biosensors & electronic health records

Clinicians need to prepare for the brave new world of digital medicine. Having acquired decades of experience with "real-world" challenges in their specialty, experienced health professionals stand in good stead as mediators between the technological industry and patients' needs and desires. We should be the ones providing this link in order to protect the interests of patients from inappropriate use of digital technology developed by PHD scientists without the benefit of prolonged interaction with patients. While we face the looming prospect of digital technology one day replacing the role of human doctors, experienced physicians should meanwhile embrace our intermediary role in helping scientists perfect their scientific developments while guiding patients on the use of digital technologies for the betterment of their health. For the benefit of patients, we should seek to keep abreast with digital medicine and not be overwhelmed by the technological tide or leave clinical decision-making solely between patients and tech providers. Unlike technologists and their machines, we as physicians have to a vow to keep – to always put our patients' best interests first.

2. Knowledge transfer during pandemic

COPD is one major disease that is multifactorial in pathogenesis and affects multiple bodily systems in such ways that multi-disciplinary collaboration is inevitable and often essential in delivering optimal care to its sufferers. At the beginning of a new decade when the world is ravaged by an unforeseen pandemic caused by the Coronavirus COVID-19, alliance of stake-holders in COPD is more essential than ever before. The reliance on technology in order to reduce physical human-to-human contact can either prove to be a boon or bane to closer cooperation to improve patient care. As the world grapples with an unwelcome novel lung infection, we cannot afford to ignore the incessant impact of a disease that continues to kills more people annually than all respiratory tract infections combined (inclusive of those related to coronavirus COVID-19, accurate at the time of writing). Knowledge transfer is imperative in fighting any disease new or old and sharing essential medical information quickly is crucial.

It is time for a new paradigm in tackling the age-old disease of COPD. No longer can stake-holders afford to research or treat this disorder in the isolation of 'ivory-tower' institutions. The expected shift in the locus of disease burden to the Majority World urgently requires contextualization of medical progress to suit local environment and habits [3]. Continuing contributions from international intelligentsia and academic sources will be helpful in developing a wider perspective of the approach to this common global disease, as well as provide clinicians everywhere an updated reference for the management of this malady.

Author details

Kian-Chung Ong
Mount Elizabeth Medical Centre, Singapore

*Address all correspondence to: dr@chestmed.com.sg

References

[1] GBD Chronic Respiratory Disease Collaborators. Lancet Respir Med. 2020;8:585-596

[2] GOLD 2020 Report. Available at: https://goldcopd.org/wp-content/uploads/2019/12/GOLD-2020-FINAL-ver1.2-03Dec19_WMV.pdf. Accessed: August 2020.

[3] Cafiero DE, et al. The Global Economic Burden of Noncommunicable Diseases. 2011, World Economic Forum: Geneva.

Chapter 2

Chronic Obstructive Pulmonary Disease Related to Wood and Other Biomass Smoke: A Different Phenotype or Specific Diseases?

Carlos A. Torres-Duque, Felipe Severiche-Bueno and Mauricio González-García

Abstract

Around 41% of the world's population continue using solid fuels, including wood and other types of biomass, for cooking or heating their homes. Long-term indoor exposure to wood smoke, and biomass smoke in general, is a risk factor for developing chronic obstructive pulmonary disease (COPD). In some regions of the world, biomass exposure is a more frequent cause of COPD than exposure to cigarette smoke. Recently it has been described notable differences between COPD associated with wood smoke (WS-COPD) and that caused by tobacco smoking (TS-COPD): significantly less emphysema and more airway inflammation in WS-COPD. Recognizing these differences, some authors have suggested that WS-COPD should be considered a new COPD phenotype. This chapter summarizes the differences between WS-COPD and TS-COPD. The information about the characteristics of COPD caused by other types of biomass fuels, different from wood, is very scarce. Accepting that the smoke derived from wood burning and tobacco smoking have some differences (etiology), the inhalation patterns are different (pathogenesis) and the physiopathological mechanisms they induce may also differ, we analyze if the disease caused by indoor chronic exposure to wood smoke should be considered as another COPD phenotype or a distinct nosological entity.

Keywords: chronic obstructive pulmonary disease (COPD), wood smoke, biomass, tobacco, phenotype, emphysema, chronic bronchitis, bronchial anthracofibrosis, indoor air pollution

1. Introduction

Solid and biomass fuels are the most important global environmental risk factor. Around 41% of the world's population, over 2.8 billion people, particularly in developing countries, still use solid fuels, whether coal or biomass (wood, vegetable remains and dung), for cooking or heating their homes [1, 2]. In some countries, these fuels are the main source of energy for over 70% of the rural population. In countries where migration from rural areas to cities is high, the population of urban dwellers over the age of 40 years frequently has a significant history of exposure to biomass fuels. One example is Colombia, where 39% of the population over 40 years of age living in the five main cities had cooked using wood as fuel for more than 10 years before relocating [3].

Between 1980 and 2010, the population exposed to household air pollution (HAP) increased from 333 million to 646 million in sub-Saharan Africa and from 162 million to 190 million in the eastern Mediterranean. In south-east Asia, it remained stable during the same period at around 1 billion people [1].

Biomass fuels are usually burnt in open fires and inefficient traditional cook-stoves, often in poorly ventilated cooking spaces, resulting in indoor high levels of air pollutants including carbon monoxide (CO) and particulate matter (PM). The people most exposed are women who are routinely responsible for cooking and their young children [4].

HAP is responsible for nearly 5% of the global disease burden, making it globally the single most important environmental risk factor [5]. In 2017, it has been estimated that HAP contributed to 1.8 million (95% CI, 1.1–2.7) deaths and 60.9 million (95% CI, 34.6–93.3) disability-adjusted life-years (DALYs) globally [6]. Respiratory disease was the leading cause of these deaths and DALYs attributable to HAP accounting for 38% of all deaths (0.7 million [0.4–1.0]) and 75% of all DALYs (45.7 million [26.8–68.8] [6]. Among the premature deaths related to HAP, 20% are due to chronic obstructive pulmonary disease (COPD) [2].

Biomass fuels and COPD. Several systematic reviews, meta-analyses and reviews of evidence confirm that individuals chronically exposed to solid fuels at home have a higher risk of developing COPD [6–13]. In addition, people chronically exposed to biomass smoke also have a high risk of chronic bronchitis [10, 14, 15]. The pooled analysis of the Pathak's study [7] showed that, globally, exposure to indoor air pollution due to solid biomass fuels increased risk of COPD by 2.65 (95% CI, 2.13–3.31) and chronic bronchitis by 2.89 (95% CI, 2.18–3.82) times more compared to non-biomass fuels. The risk of COPD was higher in Africa region (odds ratio [OR]: 3.19), Asia (OR: 2.88), South America (OR: 2.15), Europe (OR: 2.30) and North America (OR: 2.14). This distribution confirms that although the risk is higher in developing regions [16], the high risk is also present in developed countries, as some studies have shown [17, 18].

In some highly populated countries, like India and China, the exposure to biomass smoke is a significant risk factor for COPD, mainly in women living in rural zones [15, 19–24]. In some areas of India and China, this exposure is the most important risk factor of COPD [20–22, 25–30]. In Latin America, the PREPOCOL [3], the CRONICAS [31] and the PUMA [32] studies have confirmed that the use of biomass fuels, frequently wood, for cooking is a significant and independent risk factor for COPD, stronger in women from rural areas.

Although the risk of COPD from long-term indoor exposure to biomass fuels is particularly high in women [23, 33–36], a population study (n = 5539) showed that, after adjusting for age, smoking, educational level and occupational exposure, men exposed to wood smoke for more than 10 years had a higher risk of COPD (OR: 1.50) [37]. The risk of COPD increases significantly with the length of exposure to wood smoke and with simultaneous exposure to tobacco smoke [37].

This evidence supports that HAP from burning solid fuels, including biomass, is the biggest worldwide risk factor for COPD [38–40]. However, the prevalence of biomass-related COPD has not been precisely defined. The PREPOCOL study found a prevalence of 6.7% in people exposed to wood smoke and not to cigarette smoke compared to 7.8% in people exposed to cigarette smoke and not to wood smoke [37]. In rural Puno, Peru, daily use of biomass fuel for cooking among women was associated with COPD (prevalence ratio: 2.22, 95% CI: 1.02–4.81) and the population attributable risk of COPD due to daily exposure to biomass fuel smoke was 55% [31].

Some populational studies, however, found no association between exposure to biomass fuels and COPD [41, 42]. Most of the people evaluated in these studies lived near sea level, where cooking is usually done outdoors or with better ventilation. In contrast, many of the studies which document this association have included areas situated at high or intermediary altitudes, where, due to low temperatures, cooking is done all year round inside poorly ventilated homes as it occurs in winter in regions that have seasons. There is lack of standardization of questionnaires or other tools for evaluating the exposure to biomass smoke derived from cooking or heating. A recent study, from Kyrgyzstan, evaluated the prevalence of COPD associated with indoor contamination at different altitudes and found a higher prevalence of COPD at high altitude versus at low altitude (36.7% vs. 10.4%; $p < 0.001$) associated with exposure to a greater indoor contamination at high altitude [43].

2. Differences between WS-COPD and TS-COPD

Although the risk of COPD has been proven for all types of biomass fuels, studies which best characterize COPD due to this type of exposure have focused on COPD caused by inhalation of wood smoke (WS-COPD). Therefore, this chapter also focuses on the differences of WS-COPD and TS-COPD.

Core differences. A growing body of evidence supports that WS-COPD, unlike TS-COPD, is predominantly and markedly a disease of the airways with mild or minimum emphysema [44–54]. Although recent publications have focused on the compromise of the small airways in biomass COPD [46, 50, 52], different from TS-COPD, in WS-COPD there is also a notorious compromise of the central airway due to carbon deposition (bronchial anthracofibrosis) with plaque formation and reduction in the caliber of the lobar bronchi [55–57]. In addition to this fundamental pathological difference between WS-COPD and TS-COPD, there are many other differences that we summarize in **Table 1** and review it below.

Demographic differences. Women and their children are the most exposed population to indoor air pollution from biomass fuels because of women are usually responsible for cooking meals, particularly in developing countries, spending several hours a day in frequently poor ventilated kitchens, and keeping their children close to them [4, 16, 23, 30, 58, 59].

Most of the studies show that women with WS-COPD are consistently shorter in height and have higher body mass index (BMI) than women with TS-COPD [37, 44, 49, 54, 60–66]. There is not a clear explanation for this difference. In general, women with WS-COPD were born and have lived in rural areas as their ancestry, while women with TS-COPD have lived in urban areas for many years and many of them have urban ancestry. Therefore, it is possible that some ethnic, nutritional and socioeconomics conditions could be part of the explanation of the difference, but there is not consistent information about this.

Moreover, women with WS-COPD are older, suggesting that patients with this type of exposure need more time to develop the disease or are diagnosed later [30, 37, 44, 51, 61, 63–65, 67].

Clinical differences. Several studies have shown a high frequency of respiratory symptoms (cough, expectoration, and dyspnea) and chronic bronchitis in subjects exposed to biomass smoke [9, 10, 14, 61]. However, comparative studies between WS-COPD and TS-COPD have found no consistent differences. Some studies show that symptoms, not only cough and phlegm but dyspnea, are more frequent or have more impact in WS-COPD than TS-COPD [48, 61, 68, 69] but other not [63, 65, 70]. Rhonchus and wheezing are more frequent in WS-COPD [68].

Characteristics	WS-COPD	TS-COPD
Demographic data		
Sex	Predominantly women	Predominantly men
Age	Higher	Lower
Height	Lower	Higher
BMI	Higher	Lower
Clinical characteristics		
Cough and expectoration	Very common	Common
Chronic bronchitis	Common	Common
Rhonchus and wheezing	Common	Less common
Lung function tests		
$PaCO_2$	Higher (some studies)	Less high
PaO_2 and SaO_2	Lower	Less low
Obstruction (FEV_1/FVC reduced)	Mild	More severe
Reduced FEV_1	Lower	Higher
Bronchial hyperresponsiveness	Higher	Lower
DLco and DLco/VA	Normal or mildly reduced	More reduced
Radiography-tomography		
Emphysema	Uncommon and mild	Common and more severe
Bronchial thickening	Common	Less common
Bronchiectasis	Common	Uncommon
Atelectasis	Common	Uncommon
Histology		
Emphysema	Mild	More severe
Anthracosis	Common	Less common
Airway fibrosis	Common	Less common
Thickening of arteriole intima	Common	Less common
Outcomes and clinical phenotypes		
Pulmonary hypertension	More common	Less common
Quality of life	Symptoms and activities more compromised or similar	Similar or symptoms and activities less compromised
Survival	Similar after adjusting for age. Less after adjusting for age	Similar
Exacerbator phenotype	Similar	Similar
Asthma-COPD overlap phenotype	More common	Less common
Emphysema phenotype	Uncommon	More common

WS: wood smoke; TS: tobacco smoke; BMI: body mass index; DL_{CO}: carbon monoxide diffusing capacity; FEV_1: forced expiratory volume in 1 second; FVC: forced vital capacity; $PaCO_2$: carbon dioxide arterial pressure; PaO_2: oxygen arterial pressure; SaO_2: oxygen saturation; VA: alveolar volume.

Table 1.
Differences between wood smoke COPD and tobacco smoke COPD.

The greater bronchial compromise in WS-COPD documented in several publications which use functional and tomographic evaluations supports the studies which show more frequent cough, expectoration, rhonchus and wheezing in WS-COPD.

Differences in quality of life. Using the Saint George's Hospital Questionnaire, Camp *et al*. found worse symptoms and more impaired activity indices in women with WS-COPD [48]. González-Garcia *et al.*, in 138 women with COPD, showed that, at the same degree of obstruction, women with WS-COPD had a worse health status (poorer quality of life and worse dyspnea) than those with TS-COPD, without differences in comorbidities (**Figure 1**) [68]. Some studies have not shown differences in quality of life between these two groups of patients [65].

Differences in lung function. Airflow obstruction, both overall and adjusted by age, is milder [37, 48, 54, 60–63, 65] and the FEV_1 decline is slower and more homogeneous in WS-COPD [54, 62] than in TS-COPD. Ocakli *et al.* described a more significant compromise of FVC with higher FEV1/FVC ratio in people with COPD related to biomass smoke suggesting restrictive ventilatory alteration, but lung volumes were not measured [71]. The chronic airflow limitation in patients with WS-COPD is possibly due not only to the small airways compromise [46, 50, 52, 54], but to anthracofibrosis of the large airways [55–57].

A recent study, aimed to evaluate the lung volumes and the resistance and conductance of the airways using plethysmograhy, showed that residual volumes (RV),

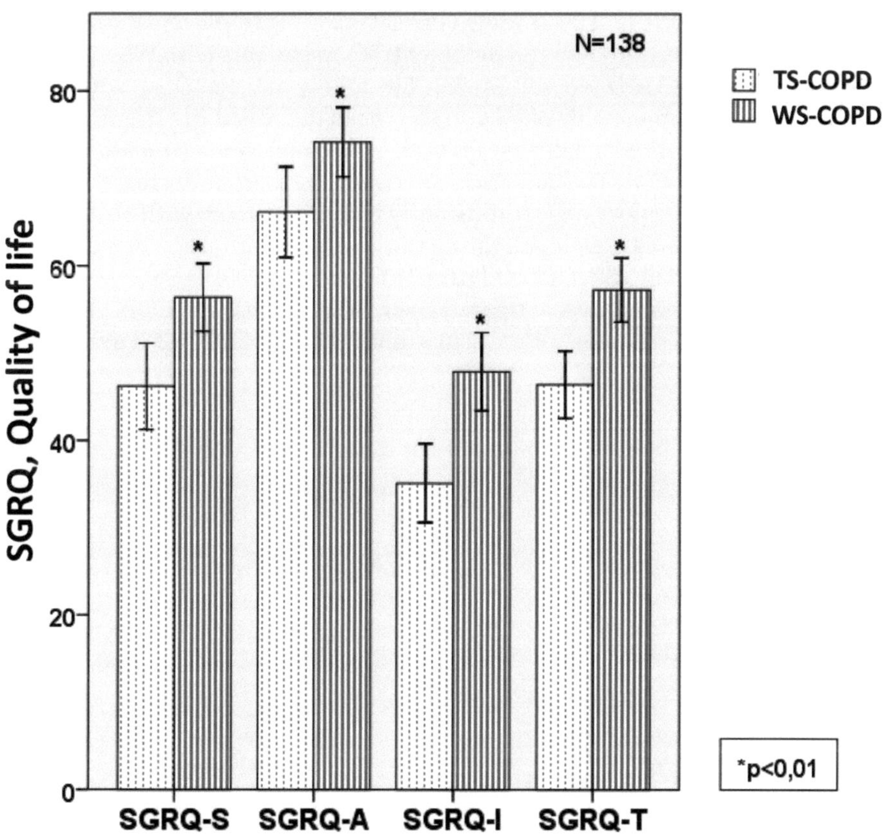

Figure 1.
Quality of life. Comparison between WS-COPD and TS-COPD. *WS-COPD: wood-smoke COPD; TS-COPD: tobacco smoke COPD. SGRQ: Saint George Respiratory Questionnaire. S: Symptoms; A: Activity; I: Impact; T: Total. From: González-García M, et al. Arch Bronconeumol. 2014; 50 (ALAT congress): 59 (ref. 68).*

total lung capacities (TLC) and RV/TLC ratios were significantly increased among both TS-COPD and non-smoking COPD (including biomass smoke COPD) subjects compared to healthy subjects ($p < 0.0001$), with no differences between the two COPD groups [54]. The same study showed that patients with COPD related to biomass smoke had significantly higher airway resistance (sRaw values) than TS-COPD patients ($p = 0.005$) and significantly lower conductance (sGaw values) in biomass COPD than in TS-COPD ($p = 0.010$) [54].

Some studies have showed that carbon dioxide arterial pressure ($PaCO_2$) is higher (lower ventilation) and oxygen arterial pressure (PaO_2) and oxygen hemoglobin saturation (SaO_2) are lower in WS-COPD than in TS-COPD [48, 61, 62, 65, 69]. Interestingly, Olloquequi *et al*. described that COPD patients who have had mixed exposure to tobacco smoke as well as biomass smoke had lower oxygen saturation than those who were exposed only to cigarette smoke or biomass smoke [72]. The lower oxygenation rates observed in WS-COPD may be explained by the compromise of the small airways and/or by hypoventilation. It remains to be determined if the higher BMI in these patients, most of whom are women over 50 years of age, is involved in this behavior.

One of most consistent differences between WS-COPD and TS-COPD is the significantly lower compromise of the diffusion capacity (DL_{CO}) in WS-COPD. DL_{CO} and DL_{CO}/alveolar volume (DL_{CO}/VA) ratio are normal or mildly altered in WS-COPD patients compared to TS-COPD patients, in who these parameters are significantly reduced [49, 60, 61], and occurs at all levels of COPD severity (**Figure 2A** and **B**) [61]. This finding correlates well with the lower grade of emphysema found on computed tomography (CT) in patients with WS-COPD in comparison with TS-COPD [48, 49, 54, 73]. The mildly reduced DL_{CO} with normal DL_{CO}/VA found in women with WS-COPD has been described in patients with significantly compromised small airways with little emphysema (pseudophysiological emphysema) [74]. The correlation between the level of decrease of FEV_1 and the level of DL_{CO} reduction is significantly better in women with TS-COPD than in those with WS-COPD, highlighting the greater contribution of emphysema to airflow obstruction in TS-COPD (**Figure 3**) [61].

Differences in bronchial hyperresponsiveness. Women with WS-COPD have greater bronchial hyperresponsiveness than women with TS-COPD (**Figure 4**) [64].

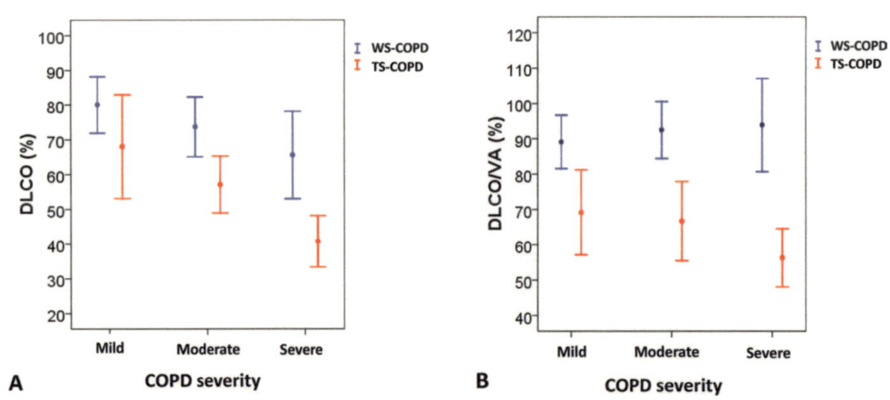

Figure 2.
Comparison of diffusion capacity between WS-COPD and TS-COPD according to degree of obstruction. *A. DL_{CO} (%) and B. DL_{CO}/VA (%). In TS-COPD, DL_{CO} and DL_{CO}/VA are more significantly compromised than in WS-COPD. DL_{CO}/VA is normal in WS-COPD at all levels of severity. WS: wood smoke; TS: tobacco smoke; DL_{CO}: carbon monoxide diffusing capacity; VA: alveolar volume.From: González-García M, et al. Acta Med Colomb. 2004; 29: 17–25 (Ref. 61).*

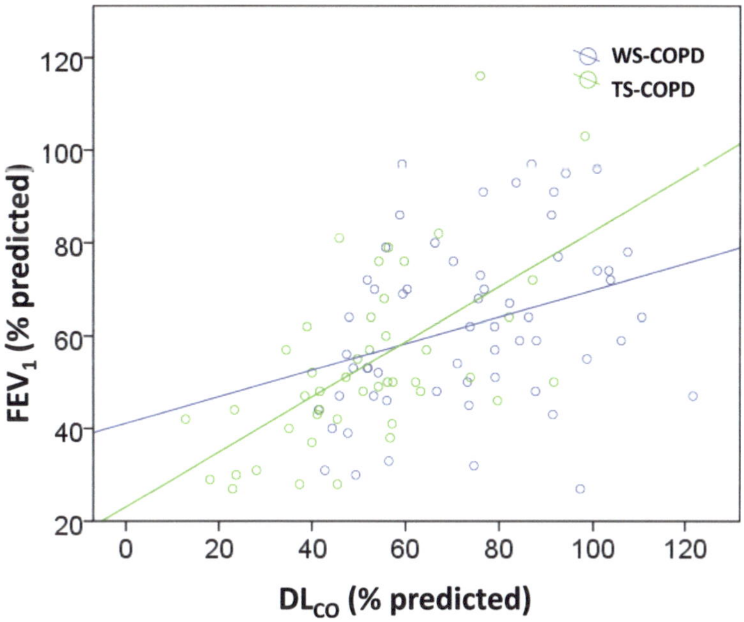

Figure 3.
Correlation between FEV_1 (%) and DL_{CO} by exposure. *Greater correlation is observed between FEV_1 and DL_{CO} in TS-COPD ($P < .001$, $r = 0.599$) than in WS-COPD ($P = .014$, $r = 0.320$). WS: Wood smoke; TS: Tobacco smoke; DL_{CO}: carbon monoxide diffusing capacity; FEV_1: forced expiratory volume in 1 s.From: González-García M, et al. Acta Med Colomb. 2004; 29: 17–25 (ref. 61).*

This finding could be correlated to the higher frequency of the asthma-COPD overlap phenotype described in biomass-related COPD [63].

Differences in exercise tolerance. Some studies which included the 6-minute walking test found no significant differences in distances walked between patients with WS-COPD and TS-COPD [48, 65, 68]. However, the study carried out by Zhao *et al.* found that patients exposed to biomass smoke walked fewer meters in the 6-minute walk than those with TS-COPD [46].

Tomography and histological differences. Patients with WS-COPD have consistently less emphysema and more airway changes (bronchial and peribronchial thickening and fibrosis, bronchiectasis, segmental and laminar subsegmental atelectasis, mosaic perfusion pattern, parenchymal bands) than patients with TS-COPD on both chest tomography and histological studies [48–50, 52, 60, 69, 73] (**Figure 5**). Bronchial and lung biopsies from patients with WS-COPD show significant inflammation and thickening of the bronchial wall, mainly of its basal membrane, squamous cell metaplasia with a remarkable anthracotic pigment deposition in the bronchi and pulmonary interstitium [60, 75–77].

Differences in the distribution of clinical phenotypes. Golpe *et al.* evaluated the frequency of clinical phenotypes defined by the 2014 Spanish COPD guidelines [78] in patients with COPD caused by biomass or tobacco smoke. They found a greater frequency of emphysema phenotype in TS-COPD and a more common asthma-COPD overlap phenotype in biomass COPD, but the difference disappeared after adjusting for sex [63]. These differences fit perfectly with the findings of the studies reported so far in this chapter. No difference was found in the frequencies of chronic bronchitis or exacerbator phenotypes [63].

Differences in pulmonary hypertension. Sertogullarindan *et al.* found that pulmonary hypertension (PH) on echocardiography was more common in WS-COPD than in TS-COPD patients [79]. In previous studies, our group, based

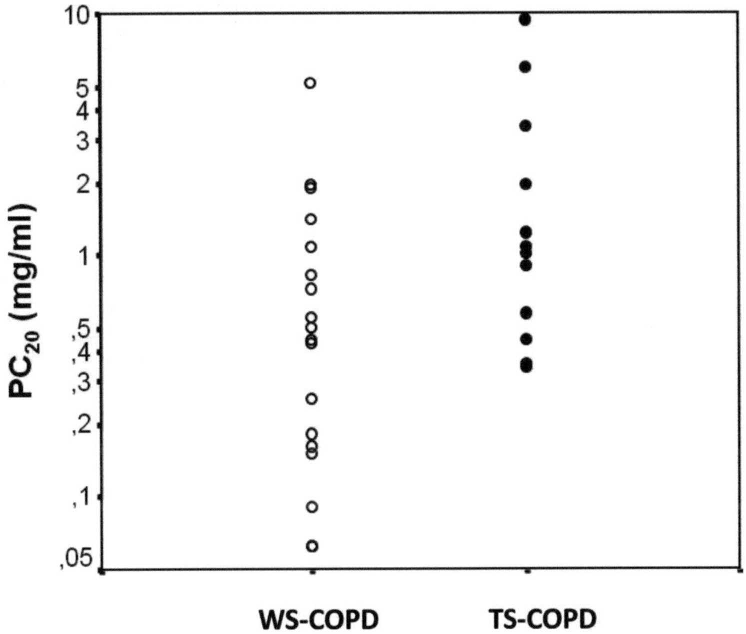

Figure 4.
Bronchial hyperresponsiveness evaluated by PC20 by exposure. *PC20: methacholine concentration causing ≥ 20% reduction in FEV_1. White circles: WS-COPD; black circles: TS-COPD. PC20 geometric mean: WS-COPD versus TS-COPD: 0.39 (0.06–5.13) versus 1.24 (0.34–9.39), P = .028. WS: wood smoke; TS: tobacco smoke. From: Gonzalez-Garcia M, et al. Int J Chron Obstruct Pulmon Dis. 2012; 7: 367–373 (Ref. 64).*

on radiographic evaluation, suggested the same higher frequency of PH in patients with severe WS-COPD [61], and Sandoval *et al.* showed a high rate of PH and cor pulmonale among patients with long-term domestic exposure to wood smoke [80]. It has been posed that the PH observed in WS-COPD could be associated not only to airflow obstruction and hypoxemia, but to a direct inflammatory effect of the inhaled smoke. It has been described that mice exposed to biomass exhibited more perivascular inflammation than those exposed to cigarette smoke [81].

Differences in the frequency of bronchial anthracofibrosis. The incidence of bronchial anthracofibrosis and its severity in individuals exposed to wood smoke or tobacco smoke has not been evaluated in prospective studies, and no differences are known. However, marked anthracofibrosis is commonly encountered in the airway of subjects exposed to wood smoke [16, 55–57], sometimes accompanied by bronchial stenosis, and it seems more frequent and severe than in tobacco smoke exposed. A significant proportion of these patients have chronic airflow limitation and meet the functional criteria of COPD [55] possibly due to the small airways compromise aggravated by anthracofibrotic central airway stenosis. It is currently impossible to ascertain if bronchial anthracofibrosis is another feature of WS-COPD that appears more commonly and in a more severe form than in TS-COPD, or if it is a specific entity accompanied by obstruction.

Differences in survival and frequency of exacerbations. After adjusting for age, sex, and disease severity, no differences have been found in survival between WS-COPD and TS-COPD [65, 82].

Recently, Cho *et al.*, among 1033 patients with COPD, have shown that patients with COPD associated with biomass smoke and those with COPD associated with tobacco smoke had a similar risk of exacerbations [67], confirming previous observations [63].

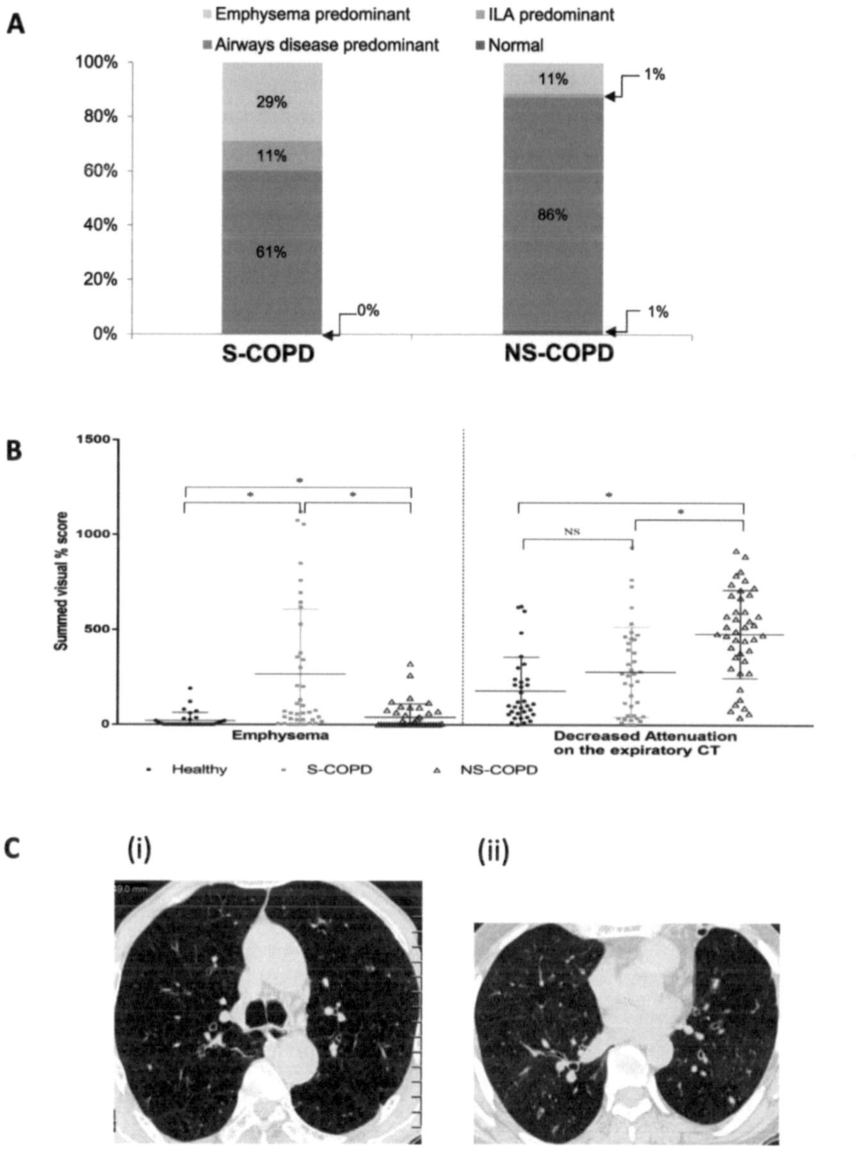

Figure 5.
Tomographic differences between smoking and non-smoking COPD*. Differences between smoker COPD (S-COPD) (n = 38) and non-smoker COPD (NS-COPD) (n = 70) on inspiratory-expiratory high resolution computerized tomography (HRCT) imaging (A) Showing HRCT classification of smoker and non-smoker COPD, including airway disease (black bars), emphysema (open bars) and interstitial lung abnormality (ILA) predominance (gray bars); (B) dot plot for emphysema and decreased attenuation of expiratory CT in S-COPD (■) and NS=COPD (△) compared to healthy subjects (●), where bars indicate median and interquartile rages and * p < 0.05, (C) Representative HRCT images of Smoker-COPD showing extensive centrilobular emphysema in the upper lobes and non-smoker COPD showing generalized decreased attenuation and some bronchial wall thickening. From: Salvi SS, et al. phenotypic comparison between smoking and non-smoking chronic obstructive pulmonary disease. Respiratory Research. 2020; 21: 50 [64].*

Differences in inflammatory profile and pathophysiological ways. It is expected that the greater airway inflammatory involvement and the lower rate of emphysema in biomass COPD, including WS-COPD, compared to TS-COPD have an etiological, pathogenic and physiopathological basis. However, although there is a growing information about the pathogenic mechanisms in COPD due to biomass smoke exposure [83], it is not clear what are the reasons explaining its differences with TS-COPD. Some studies have focused on looking for differences in the type of inflammation and the proteolytic activity, and recently the gene expression.

The exposure to biomass smoke induces pulmonary macrophages and mononuclear and polynuclear cells to generate numerous inflammatory mediators, including interleukin-6 (IL-6), interleukin-8 (IL-8), monocyte chemoattractant protein 1 (MCP-1), macrophage inflammatory protein 2 (MIP2) and tumoral necrosis factor (TNF) [83, 84]. These can generate a second wave of mediators that include enzymes, such as matrix metalloproteinase 9 (MMP-9) and matrix metalloproteinase 12 (MMP-12) involved in proteolysis and tissue remodeling typical of COPD. A recent study explored differences in chemokine and cytokine concentrations among biomass-COPD versus TS-COPD and exposed controls without COPD. The author identified CCL27 and CXCL13 as putative, plausibly homeostatic/protective biomarkers for biomass COPD [85].

Golpe *et al*. found that serum IL-6, IL-8, IL-5 were significantly higher in TS-COPD patients than in biomass COPD without differences in serum IL-13, periostin, surfactant protein-P, TNF-α, IgE, erythrocyte sedimentation rate, C-reactive protein and fibrinogen [86]. The level of exhaled nitric oxide (FeNO) was higher in biomass COPD (39.0 ± 14.6 ppb) than in TS-COPD (27.6 ± 16.3 ppb); although the difference did not reach the statistical significance level, it was borderline (p: 0.056) and it could be related to a small sample size [86].

A study by Solleiro-Villavicencio *et al*., done in women with COPD and healthy controls, found that IL-4 and T_H2 cells were significantly higher in biomass COPD than in TS-COPD [87]. Frequency of T_H17 cells in patients with TS-COPD was significantly higher than in patients with biomass COPD. They suggested that a T_H2 cytokine inflammatory profile could predominate in biomass COPD [87]. Although the majority the authors have not found differences in blood eosinophils counts between biomass COPD and TS-COPD, Fernandes *et al*., using a cutoff of ≥3%, found more frequent sputum eosinophilia in biomass COPD than in TS-COPD [88]. In the same way of the responses T_H2, Olloquequi *et al*. found higher levels of total IgE in patients with biomass smoke COPD than in TS-COPD (**Figure 6**) [72].

It seems clear that the development and clinical course of COPD depend on an interaction between genetic and environmental factors. The gene regulation and expression are fundamentally involved in the pathophysiology of COPD and it is known that microRNAs (miRNAs) participate in the control of post-transcriptional regulation in TS-COPD. Recently, Velasco-Torres *et al*. have described the differential role of miR-34a (downregulated) [89] and of the axis miR-22 - histone deacetylase activity (HDAC4) – IL-17 [90]. This axis has been linked to the development of emphysema in rats. Serum miR-22-3p was downregulated in biomass COPD-BS relative to COPD-TS. In contrast, the concentration of HDAC4 was higher in biomass and exhibited a significant positive correlation with DL_{CO}% [90]. This mechanism could be involved in the lower expression of emphysema in WS-COPD.

In summary, inflammation in biomass COPD, including WS-COPD, could be different from that in TS-COPD with a possible predominance of T_H2 profile, and the lower generation of emphysema could be related to a particular and different response to biomass smoke.

Differences in therapeutic interventions. Almost all the studies on pharmacological interventions in COPD supporting clinical guidelines and strategies [91] have been done in developed countries and use the exposure to tobacco smoke as inclusion criteria. So, the derived evidence could not be extrapolated to other causes of COPD. Taking into account the different type of inflammation, higher bronchial hyperresponsiveness and higher frequency of the asthma-COPD overlap phenotype, it is expected a benefit role of inhaled corticosteroids. To our best knowledge, there is only one study in a small sample of patients that showed better results in

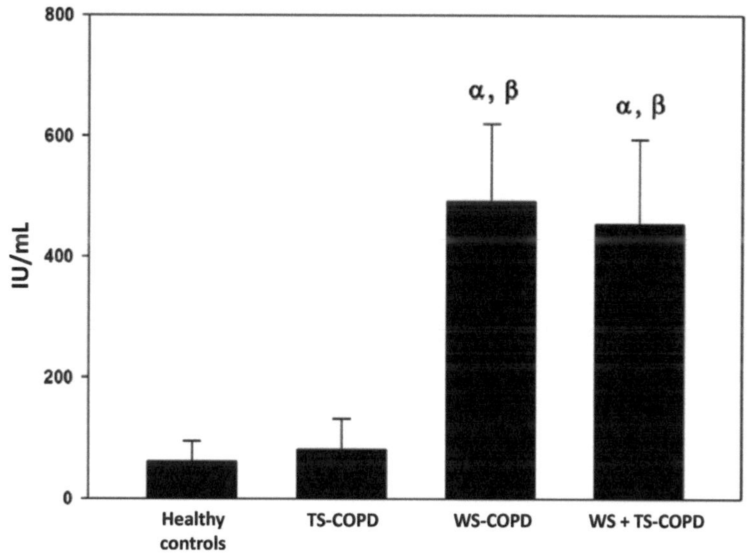

Figure 6.
IgE levels in COPD due to tobacco smoke, wood smoke or both. *α: Different from control subjects ($p < 0.05$). β: Different from TS COPD group ($p < 0.05$). TS: Tobacco smoke; WS: Wood smoke. From: Olloquequi J, et al. Respiratory Research (2018) 19:13 [72].*

reducing the exacerbation frequency and improving lung function in patients with WS-COPD with the use of ICS [92]. So, there is a lack of information regarding the efficacy and safety of pharmacological interventions in patients with WS-COPD, particularly on the potential benefits of the use of ICS in these patients.

3. COPD related to biomass fuels different from wood smoke

Biomass fuels used for cooking include mainly wood, charcoal, agricultural residues, and animal dung. The composition of these types of biomass and the smoke derived from burning it significantly differ [93]. There is growing information about the different animal and human responses to the exposures to different kind of the biomass fuels. As we have presented in this chapter, probably the most studied biomass smoke and the responses to its inhalation is wood [94, 95]. Animal manure contains greater diversity and greater quantities of microorganisms and the inflammatory response could be different [81, 96, 97]. Dung biomass smoke [96] activates inflammatory responses in human epithelial cells from airways. Cow dung exposure, but not wood smoke exposure, mediated a measurable increase in non-tipeable *Haemophilus influenzae* adhesion to airway epithelial cells.

Most of the epidemiologic, systematic reviews and meta-analysis group these types of fuels as the generic term "biomass" studies. The distribution of the types of biomass fuels used for cooking differ depending on the country and region. In certain regions, wood or wood and charcoal are the only or most used fuel but in other ones it could predominate animal dung or agricultural residues. One study in Tanzania shows that 99.5% of participants had exposure to biomass: 92.4% used wood, 14.9% used charcoal, 1.5% used crop residues and 0.6% used animal dung for cooking and heating purposes [98].

Studies that have characterized COPD, this means that have described the clinical, functional, radiographic and histopathological characteristics, have been done in wood smoke exposed, and those that have grouped patients under "biomass" exposed or "non-smokers" have included mainly people exposed to wood smoke. Therefore, it is possible that the COPD related to dung or crop residues be different and it is not recommendable to generalize the observations done in WS-COPD and described in this chapter to other types of biomass fuels.

4. Respiratory disease due to indoor chronic exposure to wood smoke: a different phenotype of COPD or a separable disease?

COPD is defined using a functional criterion and an unspecific exposure. So, under this term can be included a very numerous and heterogenous pathologic conditions. Accepting the weakness of the definition of COPD as a disease (it is more a syndrome), the WS-COPD (it is not sure if all type of biomass COPD) could be accepted as a phenotype of COPD. However, if we assume that etiology is different (wood smoke is not cigarette smoke), the inflammatory responses and the pathophysiologic could be different, and the clinical, functional and histopathologic expression are also different, the chronic respiratory disease due to long-term indoor exposure to wood smoke is better understood as a separate nosology entity. Most importantly the actions for prevention significantly differ and the therapeutic interventions could be also different.

Author details

Carlos A. Torres-Duque[1,2*], Felipe Severiche-Bueno[1,2] and Mauricio González-García[1,2]

1 Fundación Neumológica Colombiana, Bogotá, Colombia

2 La Sabana University (Universidad de La Sabana), Bogotá, Colombia

*Address all correspondence to: ctorres@neumologica.org

References

[1] Bonjour S, Adair-Rohani H, Wolf J, Bruce NG, Mehta S, Pruss-Ustun A, Lahiff M, Rehfuess EA, Mishra V, Smith KR. Solid fuel use for household cooking: country and regional estimates for 1980-2010. *Environmental Health Perspectives* 2013; 121: 784-790.

[2] WHO. World Health Organization. Household air pollution and health. 2018. https://www.who.int/news-room/fact-sheets/detail/household-air-pollution-and-health. (Accessed on: December 13, 2020). 2018.

[3] Caballero A, Torres-Duque CA, Jaramillo C, Bolivar F, Sanabria F, Osorio P, Orduz C, Guevara DP, Maldonado D. Prevalence of COPD in five Colombian cities situated at low, medium, and high altitude (PREPOCOL study). *Chest* 2008; 133: 343-349.

[4] Amegah AK, Jaakkola JJK. Household air pollution and the sustainable development goals. *Bulletin of the World Health Organization* 2016; 94: 215-221.

[5] Smith KR, Bruce N, Balakrishnan K, Adair-Rohani H, Balmes J, Chafe Z, Dherani M, Hosgood HD, Mehta S, Pope D, Rehfuess E. Millions dead: how do we know and what does it mean? Methods used in the comparative risk assessment of household air pollution. *Annual Review of Public Health* 2014; 35: 185-206.

[6] Lee KK, Bing R, Kiang J, Bashir S, Spath N, Stelzle D, Mortimer K, Bularga A, Doudesis D, Joshi SS, Strachan F, Gumy S, Adair-Rohani H, Attia EF, Chung MH, Miller MR, Newby DE, Mills NL, McAllister DA, Shah ASV. Adverse health effects associated with household air pollution: a systematic review, meta-analysis, and burden estimation study. *The Lancet Global Health* 2020; 8: e1427-e1434.

[7] Pathak U, Gupta NC, Suri JC. Risk of COPD due to indoor air pollution from biomass cooking fuel: a systematic review and meta-analysis. *International Journal of Environmental Health Research* 2019: 1-14.

[8] Hu G, Zhou Y, Tian J, Yao W, Li J, Li B, Ran P. Risk of COPD from exposure to biomass smoke: a metaanalysis. *Chest* 2010; 138: 20-31.

[9] Po JY, FitzGerald JM, Carlsten C. Respiratory disease associated with solid biomass fuel exposure in rural women and children: systematic review and meta-analysis. *Thorax* 2011; 66: 232-239.

[10] Kurmi OP, Semple S, Simkhada P, Smith WC, Ayres JG. COPD and chronic bronchitis risk of indoor air pollution from solid fuel: a systematic review and meta-analysis. *Thorax* 2010; 65: 221-228.

[11] Torres-Duque C, Maldonado D, Pérez-Padilla R, Ezzati M, Viegi G. Biomass fuels and respiratory diseases: a review of the evidence. *Proceedings of the American Thoracic Society* 2008; 5: 577-590.

[12] Gordon SB, Bruce NG, Grigg J, Hibberd PL, Kurmi OP, Lam KB, Mortimer K, Asante KP, Balakrishnan K, Balmes J, Bar-Zeev N, Bates MN, Breysse PN, Buist S, Chen Z, Havens D, Jack D, Jindal S, Kan H, Mehta S, Moschovis P, Naeher L, Patel A, Perez-Padilla R, Pope D, Rylance J, Semple S, Martin WJ, 2nd. Respiratory risks from household air pollution in low and middle income countries. *The Lancet Respiratory Medicine* 2014; 2: 823-860.

[13] Capistrano SJ, van Reyk D, Chen H, Oliver BG. Evidence of Biomass Smoke Exposure as a Causative Factor for the Development of COPD. *Toxics* 2017; 5.

[14] Gonzalez-Garcia M, Caballero A, Jaramillo C, Torres-Duque CA. Chronic

bronchitis: High prevalence in never smokers and underdiagnosis- A population-based study in Colombia. *Chronic Respiratory Disease* 2018: 1479972318769771.

[15] Panigrahi A, Padhi BK. Chronic bronchitis and airflow obstruction is associated with household cooking fuel use among never-smoking women: a community-based cross-sectional study in Odisha, India. *BMC Public Health* 2018; 18: 924.

[16] Siddharthan T, Grigsby MR, Goodman D, Chowdhury M, Rubinstein A, Irazola V, Gutierrez L, Miranda JJ, Bernabe-Ortiz A, Alam D, Kirenga B, Jones R, van Gemert F, Wise RA, Checkley W. Association between Household Air Pollution Exposure and Chronic Obstructive Pulmonary Disease Outcomes in 13 Low- and Middle-Income Country Settings. *American Journal of Respiratory and Critical Care Medicine* 2018; 197: 611-620.

[17] Orozco-Levi M, Garcia-Aymerich J, Villar J, Ramírez-Sarmiento A, Antó JM, Gea J. Wood smoke exposure and risk of chronic obstructive pulmonary disease. *The European Respiratory Journal* 2006; 27: 542-546.

[18] Raju S, Keet CA, Paulin LM, Matsui EC, Peng RD, Hansel NN, McCormack MC. Rural Residence and Poverty Are Independent Risk Factors for Chronic Obstructive Pulmonary Disease in the United States. *American Journal of Respiratory and Critical Care Medicine* 2019; 199: 961-969.

[19] Kalkana T, Moitra S, Jindal SK, Moitra S. Increasing burden of COPD in rural India: an example why India warrants primary healthcare reforms. *ERJ Open Research* 2016; 2: 00032-02016.

[20] McKay AJ, Mahesh PA, Fordham JZ, Majeed A. Prevalence of COPD in India: a systematic review. *Primary Care Respiratory Journal : Journal of the General Practice Airways Group* 2012; 21: 313-321.

[21] KalagoudaMahishale V, Angadi N, Metgudmath V, Lolly M, Eti A, Khan S. The Prevalence of Chronic Obstructive Pulmonary Disease and the Determinants of Underdiagnosis in Women Exposed to Biomass Fuel in India- a Cross Section Study. *Chonnam Medical Journal* 2016; 52: 117-122.

[22] Liu S, Zhou Y, Wang X, Wang D, Lu J, Zheng J, Zhong N, Ran P. Biomass fuels are the probable risk factor for chronic obstructive pulmonary disease in rural South China. *Thorax* 2007; 62: 889-897.

[23] Sana A, Somda SMA, Meda N, Bouland C. Chronic obstructive pulmonary disease associated with biomass fuel use in women: a systematic review and meta-analysis. *BMJ Open Respiratory Research* 2018; 5.

[24] Smith M, Li L, Augustyn M, Kurmi O, Chen J, Collins R, Guo Y, Han Y, Qin J, Xu G, Wang J, Bian Z, Zhou G, Peto R, Chen Z. Prevalence and correlates of airflow obstruction in ~317 000 never-smokers in China. 2014; 44: 66-77.

[25] Wang C, Xu J, Yang L, Xu Y, Zhang X, Bai C, Kang J, Ran P, Shen H, Wen F, Huang K, Yao W, Sun T, Shan G, Yang T, Lin Y, Wu S, Zhu J, Wang R, Shi Z, Zhao J, Ye X, Song Y, Wang Q, Zhou Y, Ding L, Yang T, Chen Y, Guo Y, Xiao F, Lu Y, Peng X, Zhang B, Xiao D, Chen CS, Wang Z, Zhang H, Bu X, Zhang X, An L, Zhang S, Cao Z, Zhan Q, Yang Y, Cao B, Dai H, Liang L, He J. Prevalence and risk factors of chronic obstructive pulmonary disease in China (the China Pulmonary Health [CPH] study): a national cross-sectional study. *Lancet (London, England)* 2018; 391: 1706-1717.

[26] Yang Y, Mao J, Ye Z, Li J, Zhao H, Liu Y. Risk factors of chronic obstructive pulmonary disease among adults in Chinese mainland: A systematic review and meta-analysis. *Respiratory Medicine* 2017; 131: 158-165.

[27] Zhang JJ, Smith KR. Household air pollution from coal and biomass fuels in China: measurements, health impacts, and interventions. *Environmental Health Perspectives* 2007; 115: 848-855.

[28] Zhu B, Wang Y, Ming J, Chen W, Zhang L. Disease burden of COPD in China: a systematic review. *International Journal of Chronic Obstructive Pulmonary Disease* 2018; 13: 1353-1364.

[29] The burden of chronic respiratory diseases and their heterogeneity across the states of India: the Global Burden of Disease Study 1990-2016. *The Lancet Global Health* 2018; 6: e1363-e1374.

[30] Chan KH, Kurmi OP, Bennett DA, Yang L, Chen Y, Tan Y, Pei P, Zhong X, Chen J, Zhang J, Kan H, Peto R, Lam KBH, Chen Z. Solid Fuel Use and Risks of Respiratory Diseases. A Cohort Study of 280,000 Chinese Never-Smokers. *American Journal of Respiratory and Critical Care Medicine* 2019; 199: 352-361.

[31] Jaganath D, Miranda JJ, Gilman RH, Wise RA, Diette GB, Miele CH, Bernabe-Ortiz A, Checkley W, Group CCS. Prevalence of chronic obstructive pulmonary disease and variation in risk factors across four geographically diverse resource-limited settings in Peru. *Respiratory Research* 2015; 16: 40-40.

[32] Montes de Oca M, Zabert G, Moreno D, Laucho-Contreras ME, Lopez Varela MV, Surmont F. Smoke, Biomass Exposure, and COPD Risk in the Primary Care Setting: The PUMA Study. *Respiratory Care* 2017; 62: 1058-1066.

[33] Perez-Padilla R, Regalado J, Vedal S, Pare P, Chapela R, Sansores R, Selman M. Exposure to biomass smoke and chronic airway disease in Mexican women. A case-control study. *American Journal of Respiratory and Critical Care Medicine* 1996; 154: 701-706.

[34] Regalado J, Perez-Padilla R, Sansores R, Paramo Ramirez JI, Brauer M, Pare P, Vedal S. The effect of biomass burning on respiratory symptoms and lung function in rural Mexican women. *American Journal of Respiratory and Critical Care Medicine* 2006; 174: 901-905.

[35] Dennis RJ, Maldonado D, Norman S, Baena E, Martinez G. Woodsmoke exposure and risk for obstructive airways disease among women. *Chest* 1996; 109: 115-119.

[36] Kiraz K, Kart L, Demir R, Oymak S, Gulmez I, Unalacak M, Ozesmi M. Chronic pulmonary disease in rural women exposed to biomass fumes. *Clinical and Investigative Medicine Medecine Clinique et Experimentale* 2003; 26: 243-248.

[37] Torres-Duque C, Caballero A, González-García M, Jaramillo C, Maldonado D. Chronic obstructive pulmonary disease in people exposed to Wood smoke. PREPOCOL: a population based study. *Am J Respir Crit Care Med* 2013; 187: A364.

[38] Salvi S, Barnes PJ. Is exposure to biomass smoke the biggest risk factor for COPD globally? *Chest* 2010; 138: 3-6.

[39] Mortimer K, Gordon SB, Jindal SK, Accinelli RA, Balmes J, Martin WJ, 2nd. Household air pollution is a major avoidable risk factor for cardiorespiratory disease. *Chest* 2012; 142: 1308-1315.

[40] BellouV,BelbasisL,KonstantinidisAK, Evangelou E. Elucidating the risk factors

for chronic obstructive pulmonary disease: an umbrella review of meta-analyses. *The International Journal of Tuberculosis and Lung Disease : The Official Journal of the International Union against Tuberculosis and Lung Disease* 2019; 23: 58-66.

[41] Menezes AM, Perez-Padilla R, Jardim JR, Muiño A, Lopez MV, Valdivia G, Montes de Oca M, Talamo C, Hallal PC, Victora CG. Chronic obstructive pulmonary disease in five Latin American cities (the PLATINO study): a prevalence study. *Lancet (London, England)* 2005; 366: 1875-1881.

[42] Lamprecht B, McBurnie MA, Vollmer WM, Gudmundsson G, Welte T, Nizankowska-Mogilnicka E, Studnicka M, Bateman E, Anto JM, Burney P, Mannino DM, Buist SA. COPD in never smokers: results from the population-based burden of obstructive lung disease study. *Chest* 2011; 139: 752-763.

[43] Brakema EA, Tabyshova A, Kasteleyn MJ, Molendijk E, van der Kleij R, van Boven JFM, Emilov B, Akmatalieva M, Mademilov M, Numans ME, Williams S, Sooronbaev T, Chavannes NH. High COPD prevalence at high altitude: does household air pollution play a role? *The European Respiratory Journal* 2019; 53.

[44] Pérez-Padilla R, Ramirez-Venegas A, Sansores-Martinez R. Clinical Characteristics of Patients With Biomass Smoke-Associated COPD and Chronic Bronchitis, 2004-2014. *Chronic Obstructive Pulmonary Diseases: Journal of the COPD Foundation* 2014; 1: 23-32.

[45] Torres-Duque CA, Garcia-Rodriguez MC, Gonzalez-Garcia M. Is Chronic Obstructive Pulmonary Disease Caused by Wood Smoke a Different Phenotype or a Different Entity? *Archivos de Bronconeumologia* 2016; 52: 425-431.

[46] Zhao D, Zhou Y, Jiang C, Zhao Z, He F, Ran P. Small airway disease: A different phenotype of early stage COPD associated with biomass smoke exposure. *Respirology (Carlton, Vic)* 2018; 23: 198-205.

[47] Perret JL, Abramson MJ. Biomass smoke COPD: A phenotype or a different disease? *Respirology (Carlton, Vic)* 2018; 23: 124-125.

[48] Camp PG, Ramirez-Venegas A, Sansores RH, Alva LF, McDougall JE, Sin DD, Pare PD, Muller NL, Silva CI, Rojas CE, Coxson HO. COPD phenotypes in biomass smoke- versus tobacco smoke-exposed Mexican women. *The European Respiratory Journal* 2014; 43: 725-734.

[49] Gonzalez-Garcia M, Maldonado Gomez D, Torres-Duque CA, Barrero M, Jaramillo Villegas C, Perez JM, Varon H. Tomographic and functional findings in severe COPD: comparison between the wood smoke-related and smoking-related disease. *Jornal Brasileiro de Pneumologia : Publicacao Oficial da Sociedade Brasileira de Pneumologia e Tisilogia* 2013; 39: 147-154.

[50] Fernandes L, Gulati N, Fernandes Y, Mesquita AM, Sardessai M, Lammers JJ, Mohamed Hoesein FA, Ten Hacken NHT, van den Berge M, Galban CJ, Siddiqui S. Small airway imaging phenotypes in biomass- and tobacco smoke-exposed patients with COPD. *ERJ Open Res* 2017; 3.

[51] Assad NA, Balmes J, Mehta S, Cheema U, Sood A. Chronic obstructive pulmonary disease secondary to household air pollution. *Seminars in Respiratory and Critical Care Medicine* 2015; 36: 408-421.

[52] Ramirez-Venegas A, Torres-Duque CA, Guzman-Bouilloud NE, Gonzalez-Garcia M, Sansores RH. Small airway disease in COPD associated to biomass exposure. *Revista de*

Investigacion Clinica; Organo del Hospital de Enfermedades de la Nutricion 2019; 71: 70-78.

[53] Jindal S, Jindal A. COPD in Biomass exposed nonsmokers: a different phenotype. *Expert Review of Respiratory Medicine* 2020: 1-8.

[54] Salvi SS, Brashier BB, Londhe J, Pyasi K, Vincent V, Kajale SS, Tambe S, Mandani K, Nair A, Mak SM, Madas S, Juvekar S, Donnelly LE, Barnes PJ. Phenotypic comparison between smoking and non-smoking chronic obstructive pulmonary disease. *Respiratory Research* 2020; 21: 50.

[55] Kim YJ, Jung CY, Shin HW, Lee BK. Biomass smoke induced bronchial anthracofibrosis: presenting features and clinical course. *Respiratory Medicine* 2009; 103: 757-765.

[56] Gupta A, Shah A. Bronchial anthracofibrosis: an emerging pulmonary disease due to biomass fuel exposure. *The International Journal of Tuberculosis and Lung Disease : The Official Journal of the International Union against Tuberculosis and Lung Disease* 2011; 15: 602-612.

[57] Kim H, Cha SI, Shin KM, Lim JK, Oh S, Kim MJ, Lee YD, Kim M, Lee J, Kim CH. Clinical relevance of bronchial anthracofibrosis in patients with chronic obstructive pulmonary disease exacerbation. *Tuberculosis and Respiratory Diseases* 2014; 77: 124-131.

[58] Duan JX, Cheng W, Zeng YQ, Chen Y, Cai S, Li X, Zhu YQ, Chen M, Zhou ML, Ma LB, Liu QM, Chen P. Characteristics of Patients with Chronic Obstructive Pulmonary Disease Exposed to Different Environmental Risk Factors: A Large Cross-Sectional Study. *Int J Chron Obstruct Pulmon Dis* 2020; 15: 2857-2867.

[59] Moreira M, Barbosa M, Jardim J, Queiroz M, Inácio L. Doença pulmonar obstrutiva crônica em mulheres expostas à fumaça de fogão à lenha. . *Revista da Associação Médica Brasileira* 2013; 59: 607-613.

[60] Moran-Mendoza O, Perez-Padilla JR, Salazar-Flores M, Vazquez-Alfaro F. Wood smoke-associated lung disease: a clinical, functional, radiological and pathological description. *The International Journal of Tuberculosis and Lung Disease : The Official Journal of the International Union against Tuberculosis and Lung Disease* 2008; 12: 1092-1098.

[61] González M, Páez S, Jaramillo C, Barrero M, Maldonado D. Enfermedad pulmonar obstructiva crónica (EPOC) por humo de leña en mujeres. *Acta Med Colomb* 2004; 29: 17-25.

[62] Ramirez-Venegas A, Sansores RH, Quintana-CarrilloRH,Velazquez-UncalM, Hernandez-ZentenoRJ,Sanchez-RomeroC, Velazquez-Montero A, Flores-Trujillo F. FEV1 decline in patients with chronic obstructive pulmonary disease associated with biomass exposure. *American Journal of Respiratory and Critical Care Medicine* 2014; 190: 996-1002.

[63] Golpe R, Sanjuan Lopez P, Cano Jimenez E, Castro Anon O, Perez de Llano LA. Distribution of clinical phenotypes in patients with chronic obstructive pulmonary disease caused by biomass and tobacco smoke. *Archivos de Bronconeumologia* 2014; 50: 318-324.

[64] Gonzalez-Garcia M, Torres-Duque CA, Bustos A, Jaramillo C, Maldonado D. Bronchial hyperresponsiveness in women with chronic obstructive pulmonary disease related to wood smoke. *Int J Chron Obstruct Pulmon Dis* 2012; 7: 367-373.

[65] Ramirez-Venegas A, Sansores RH, Perez-Padilla R, Regalado J, Velazquez A, Sanchez C, Mayar ME. Survival of patients with chronic

obstructive pulmonary disease due to biomass smoke and tobacco. *American Journal of Respiratory and Critical Care Medicine* 2006; 173: 393-397.

[66] Pérez-Bautista O, Montaño M, Pérez-Padilla R, Zúñiga-Ramos J, Camacho-Priego M, Barrientos-Gutiérrez T, Buendía-Roldan I, Velasco-Torres Y, Ramos C. Women with COPD by biomass show different serum profile of adipokines, incretins, and peptide hormones than smokers. *RESPIRATORY RESEARCH* 2018; 19: 239.

[67] Cho J, Lee C-H, Hwang S-s, Kim KU, Lee SH, Park HY, Park SJ, Min KH, Oh Y-M, Yoo KH, Jung K-S, on behalf of the K, Investigators K. Risk of acute exacerbations in chronic obstructive pulmonary disease associated with biomass smoke compared with tobacco smoke. *BMC Pulmonary Medicine* 2019; 19: 68.

[68] González-García M GV, Perlaza I, Casas A. Diferencias en el impacto sobre el estado de salud entre la EPOC por cigarrillo y por humo de leña. *Archivos de Bronconeumologia* 2014; 50 (Numero Especial Congreso ALAT): 59.

[69] Meneghini AC, Koenigkam-Santos M, Pereira MC, Tonidandel PR, Terra-Filho J, Cunha FQ, Menezes MBd, Vianna EO. Biomass smoke COPD has less tomographic abnormalities but worse hypoxemia compared with tobacco COPD %J Brazilian Journal of Medical and Biological Research. 2019; 52.

[70] Moreira MAC, Moraes MRd, Silva DGST, Pinheiro TF, Vasconcelos Júnior HM, Maia LFdL, Couto DVd. Estudo comparativo de sintomas respiratórios e função pulmonar em pacientes com doença pulmonar obstrutiva crônica relacionada à exposição à fumaça de lenha e de tabaco %J Jornal Brasileiro de Pneumologia. 2008; 34: 667-674.

[71] Ocakli B, Acarturk E, Aksoy E, Gungor S, Ciyiltepe F, Oztas S, Ozmen I, Agca MC, Salturk C, Adiguzel N, Karakurt Z. The impact of exposure to biomass smoke versus cigarette smoke on inflammatory markers and pulmonary function parameters in patients with chronic respiratory failure. *Int J Chron Obstruct Pulmon Dis* 2018; 13: 1261-1267.

[72] Olloquequi J, Jaime S, Parra V, Cornejo-Córdova E, Valdivia G, Agustí À, Silva O R. Comparative analysis of COPD associated with tobacco smoking, biomass smoke exposure or both. *Respiratory Research* 2018; 19: 13.

[73] Moreira MA, Barbosa MA, Queiroz MC, Teixeira KI, Torres PP, Santana Junior PJ, Montadon Junior ME, Jardim JR. Pulmonary changes on HRCT scans in nonsmoking females with COPD due to wood smoke exposure. *Jornal Brasileiro de Pneumologia : Publicacao Oficial da Sociedade Brasileira de Pneumologia e Tisilogia* 2013; 39: 155-163.

[74] Gelb AF, Zamel N, Hogg JC, Müller NL, Schein MJ. Pseudophysiologic emphysema resulting from severe small-airways disease. *American Journal of Respiratory and Critical Care Medicine* 1998; 158: 815-819.

[75] Rivera RM, Cosio MG, Ghezzo H, Salazar M, Perez-Padilla R. Comparison of lung morphology in COPD secondary to cigarette and biomass smoke. *The International Journal of Tuberculosis and Lung Disease : The Official Journal of the International Union against Tuberculosis and Lung Disease* 2008; 12: 972-977.

[76] Palacios DM, Méndez O. NeumopatÍa por humo de leña Un estudio en autopsias. *Biomédica* 1998; 18: 153-160.

[77] Restrepo J, Reyes P, de Ochoa P, Patino E. Neumoconiosis por inhalación

del humo de leña. *Acta Med Colomb* 1983; 8: 191-204.

[78] Miravitlles M, Soler-Cataluña JJ, Calle M, Molina J, Almagro P, Quintano JA, Riesco JA, Trigueros JA, Piñera P, Simón A, Rodríguez-Hermosa JL, Marco E, López D, Coll R, Coll-Fernández R, Lobo MÁ, Díez J, Soriano JB, Ancochea J. Guía española de la EPOC (GesEPOC). Actualización 2014. *Archivos de Bronconeumologia* 2014; 50: 1-16.

[79] Sertogullarindan B, Gumrukcuoglu HA, Sezgi C, Akil MA. Frequency of pulmonary hypertension in patients with COPD due to biomass smoke and tobacco smoke. *International Journal of Medical Sciences* 2012; 9: 406-412.

[80] Sandoval J, Salas J, Martinez-Guerra ML, Gómez A, Martinez C, Portales A, Palomar A, Villegas M, Barrios R. Pulmonary arterial hypertension and cor pulmonale associated with chronic domestic woodsmoke inhalation. *Chest* 1993; 103: 12-20.

[81] Mehra D, Geraghty PM, Hardigan AA, Foronjy R. A comparison of the inflammatory and proteolytic effects of dung biomass and cigarette smoke exposure in the lung. *PloS one* 2012; 7: e52889.

[82] Golpe R, Mengual-Macenlle N, Sanjuan-Lopez P, Cano-Jimenez E, Castro-Anon O, Perez-de-Llano LA. Prognostic Indices and Mortality Prediction in COPD Caused by Biomass Smoke Exposure. *Lung* 2015; 193: 497-503.

[83] Silva R, Oyarzún M, Olloquequi J. Pathogenic mechanisms in chronic obstructive pulmonary disease due to biomass smoke exposure. *Archivos de Bronconeumologia* 2015; 51: 285-292.

[84] Dutta A, Roychoudhury S, Chowdhury S, Ray MR. Changes in sputum cytology, airway inflammation and oxidative stress due to chronic inhalation of biomass smoke during cooking in premenopausal rural Indian women. *International Journal of Hygiene and Environmental Health* 2013; 216: 301-308.

[85] Vishweswaraiah S, Thimraj TA, George L, Krishnarao CS, Lokesh KS, Siddaiah JB, Larsson K, Upadhyay S, Palmberg L, Anand MP, Ganguly K. Putative Systemic Biomarkers of Biomass Smoke-Induced Chronic Obstructive Pulmonary Disease among Women in a Rural South Indian Population. *Disease Markers* 2018; 2018: 4949175.

[86] Golpe R, Martín-Robles I, Sanjuán-López P, Pérez-de-Llano L, González-Juanatey C, López-Campos JL, Arellano-Orden E. Differences in systemic inflammation between cigarette and biomass smoke-induced COPD. *Int J Chron Obstruct Pulmon Dis* 2017; 12: 2639-2646.

[87] Solleiro-Villavicencio H, Quintana-Carrillo R, Falfan-Valencia R, Vargas-Rojas MI. Chronic obstructive pulmonary disease induced by exposure to biomass smoke is associated with a Th2 cytokine production profile. *Clinical Immunology (Orlando, Fla)* 2015; 161: 150-155.

[88] Fernandes L, Rane S, Mandrekar S, Mesquita AM. Eosinophilic Airway Inflammation in Patients with Stable Biomass Smoke- versus Tobacco Smoke-Associated Chronic Obstructive Pulmonary Disease. *Journal of Health & Pollution* 2019; 9: 191209.

[89] Velasco-Torres Y, Ruiz-López V, Pérez-Bautista O, Buendía-Roldan I, Ramírez-Venegas A, Pérez-Ramos J, Falfán-Valencia R, Ramos C, Montaño M. miR-34a in serum is involved in mild-to-moderate COPD in women exposed to biomass smoke. *BMC Pulm Med* 2019; 19: 227.

[90] Velasco-Torres Y, Ruiz V, Montaño M, Pérez-Padilla R, Falfán-Valencia R, Pérez-Ramos J, Pérez-Bautista O, Ramos C. Participation of the miR-22-HDAC4-DLCO Axis in Patients with COPD by Tobacco and Biomass. *Biomolecules* 2019; 9.

[91] Vogelmeier CF, Criner GJ, Martinez FJ, Anzueto A, Barnes PJ, BourbeauJ,CelliBR,ChenR,DecramerM, Fabbri LM, Frith P, Halpin DM, Lopez Varela MV, Nishimura M, Roche N, Rodriguez-Roisin R, Sin DD, Singh D, Stockley R, Vestbo J, Wedzicha JA, Agusti A. Global Strategy for the Diagnosis, Management, and Prevention of Chronic Obstructive Lung Disease 2017 Report. GOLD Executive Summary. *American Journal of Respiratory and Critical Care Medicine* 2017; 195: 557-582.

[92] Deb A, Agarwal M, Reddy V, Kodgule R, Hemalatha V, Awasthi A, al. e. Effects of a fixed dose once-daily triple drug combination in smokers and non-smokers with COPD. . *The European Respiratory Journal* 2016; 48: PA654.

[93] Chen J, Li C, Ristovski Z, Milic A, Gu Y, Islam MS, Wang S, Hao J, Zhang H, He C, Guo H, Fu H, Miljevic B, Morawska L, Thai P, Lam YF, Pereira G, Ding A, Huang X, Dumka UC. A review of biomass burning: Emissions and impacts on air quality, health and climate in China. *Science of The Total Environment* 2017; 579: 1000-1034.

[94] Naeher LP, Brauer M, Lipsett M, Zelikoff JT, Simpson CD, Koenig JQ, Smith KR. Woodsmoke health effects: a review. *Inhalation Toxicology* 2007; 19: 67-106.

[95] Zelikoff JT, Chen LC, Cohen MD, Schlesinger RB. The toxicology of inhaled woodsmoke. *Journal of Toxicology and Environmental Health Part B, Critical Reviews* 2002; 5: 269-282.

[96] McCarthy CE, Duffney PF, Gelein R, Thatcher TH, Elder A, Phipps RP, Sime PJ. Dung biomass smoke activates inflammatory signaling pathways in human small airway epithelial cells. *American Journal of Physiology Lung Cellular and Molecular Physiology* 2016; 311: L1222-l1233.

[97] Kc R, Hyland I, Smith J, Shukla S, Hansbro P, Zosky G, Karupiah G, O'Toole R. Cow Dung Biomass Smoke Exposure Increases Adherence of Respiratory Pathogen Nontypeable Haemophilus influenzae to Human Bronchial Epithelial Cells. *Exposure and Health* 2020; 12.

[98] Magitta NwF, Walker RW, Apte KK, Shimwela MD, Mwaiselage JD, Sanga AA, Namdeo AK, Madas SJ, Salvi SS. Prevalence, risk factors and clinical correlates of COPD in a rural setting in Tanzania. 2018; 51: 1700182.

Chapter 3

Work - Related Chronic Obstructive Pulmonary Disease

Biruk Getahun and Abebe Ayalew Bekel

Abstract

Chronic obstructive pulmonary disease (COPD) is a progressive lung disease characterized by airflow obstruction and increasing breathlessness. COPD is increasing worldwide, both in developed and developing countries. The most important risk factor of developing COPD is cigarette smoking; however, occupational exposures such as vapors, gases, dusts and fumes present an important risk factor for the development of the disease, by itself and through interaction with other risk factors. The dusts from coal, stone quarries, wood, cereals and agricultural work, animal stables, textiles, and paper production that can arise in occupational environments have been regulated by the International Labor Organization and considered possible as contributors to COPD. A better understanding of these causes paves the way for effective interventions to reduce the future incidence of this unpleasant condition. Breathlessness and occupational exposures to vapors, gases, dusts and fumes were identified as the main modifiable factors associated with unemployment and poor work productivity in COPD patients.

Keywords: occupational exposures, work place, air pollutions, airflow obstruction

1. Introduction

Chronic obstructive pulmonary disease (COPD) accounts worldwide for considerable and increasing morbidity and mortality [1].

COPD is a long-term respiratory disease which is not completely reversible and is characterized by airflow obstruction. For several months, the airflow obstruction does not alter markedly and is typically progressive. COPD is mainly caused by smoking [2]. Other factors, such as harmful dust and chemicals, can also contribute to the development of COPD, especially occupational exposure [3]. People with COPD often have exacerbations when symptoms are quickly and sustainably exacerbated beyond their normal regular variation. The prevalence of COPD has major regional differences and is closely correlated with levels of deprivation. The prevalence of COPD has not decreased in recent years, unlike many other prevalent chronic illnesses [2].

Early diagnosis and treatment will help to delay the deterioration in lung function and improve the amount of time people with COPD have to enjoy an active life. COPD is treatable but not curable. In spite of having only minimal or no effect on airflow obstruction, pharmacological and other therapies can help manage symptoms and disabilities caused by COPD and improve the quality of life of the individual [1].

2. Definition and description of COPD

COPD is a progressive lung disease, characterized by airflow limitation [4]. Chronic respiratory disease is generally divided into obstructive and restrictive conditions (**Figure 1**). The Global Initiative on Obstructive Lung Disease (GOLD) has recommended that obstruction should be defined as the ratio of the forced expiratory volume in 1 s (FEV1) to forced vital capacity (FVC) of <70% (**Table 1**).

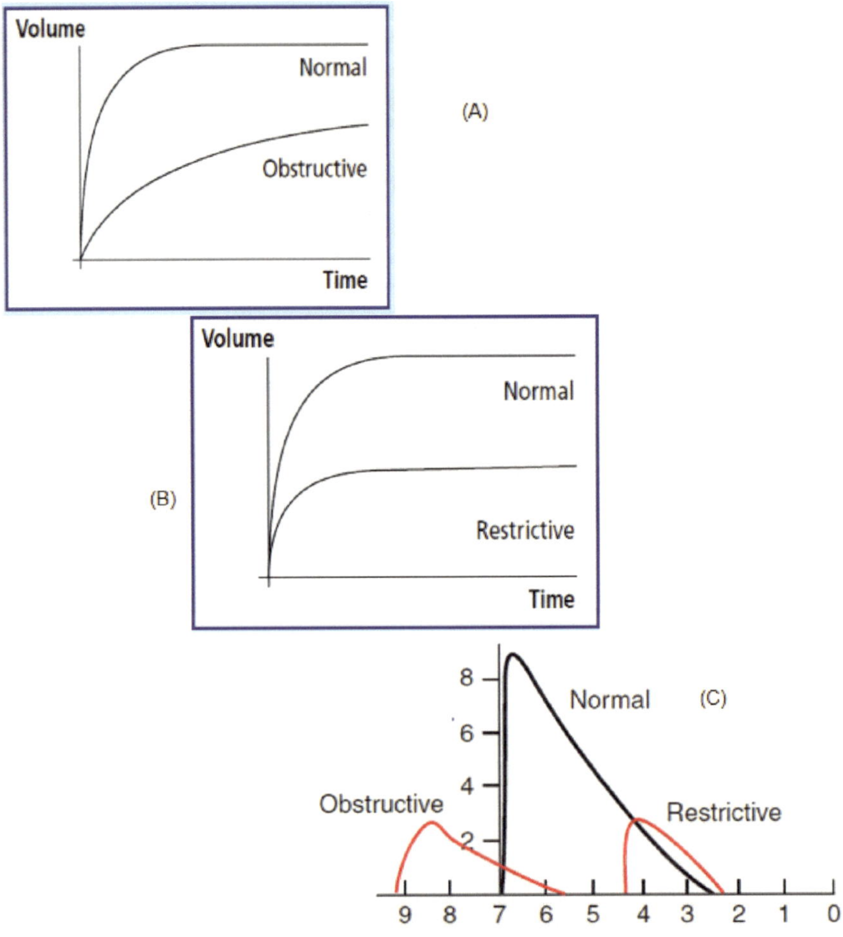

Figure 1.
Volume-time and flow-volume curves: A & B are volume – Time curves; C: Flow volume curve [5, 6].

Disease severity	GOLD staging	Spirometry criteria
Mild	GOLD 1	$FEV_1/FVC < 0.70$ $FEV_1 > 80\%$ predicted
Moderate	GOLD 2	$FEV_1/FVC < 0.70$ $50\% < FEV_1 < 80\%$ predicted
Severe	GOLD 3	$FEV_1/FVC < 0.70$ $30\% < FEV_1 < 50\%$ predicted
Very severe	GOLD 4	$FEV_1/FVC < 0.70$ $FEV_1 < 30\%$ predicted

Table 1.
Global initiative for chronic obstructive lung disease (GOLD) classification disease severity staging [4].

If any of the FVC, FEV1, PEF or FEV1/FVC are outside the normal range, the presence of ventilator abnormality can be inferred. A reduction of FEV1 would result in a low FEV1/FVC in comparison to the forced vital capacity and is characteristic of obstructive ventilator defects. The lower limit of normal for FEV_1/FVC is around 70–75% but the exact limit is dependent on age. In restrictive ventilator defect the FEV_1/FVC ratio remains normal or high (typically >70%) with a reduction in both FEV1 and FVC. A reduced FVC together with a low FEV_1/FVC ratio is a feature of a mixed ventilator defect in which a combination of both obstruction and restriction appear to be present [7, 8].

3. Occupational exposure and COPD

Associations between chronic respiratory symptoms and workplace exposures have been suggested as early as the 15th century, although documentation of the connection between 'dusty trades' and chronic bronchitis has been more prominent from the 19th century. The inconsistent definitions of COPD and unreliable measure of exposures have led to a delay in the recognition of the causal link between occupational exposures and COPD. However, over recent years strong associations have been found between particular occupational groups and exposures to vapors, gases, dusts and fumes (VGDF) and the development of COPD [4, 9].

Strong evidence implicates occupational exposures as one of the causes of COPD [4, 10, 11]. A significant part of the literature accumulated over the past two decades demonstrated the relationship between vapor, gases, dust, and fumes (VGDF) and the development of COPD. Based on a review by the American Thoracic Society (ATS) [12], and a subsequent updated review it has been estimated that approximately 15% of COPD may be attributable to workplace exposures [4]. Workers are exposed to respiratory toxicants in various occupations such as mining, manufacturing, and even office buildings, which can cause disease along the respiratory tract at any point [13, 14]. Up to 15 percent of asthma and 10 percent of lung cancer can be due to occupational exposure. Workers are exposed to a distinct and more complex spectrum of respiratory exposures in developing countries than workers in developed countries, as laws may not be as functional and environmental regulations may not be as advanced [13].

At any point along the respiratory tract, which spans the nasal cavity into the small air sacs (alveoli) in the lung tissue, disease may occur. Disease may involve the airways inside the lung itself, contributing to common diseases such as asthma and chronic obstructive pulmonary disease (COPD). There is a wide variety of exposures to airway disease, including animal and plant materials, various synthetic chemicals, metal and wood products, and irritants such as welding fumes and acid gases [13, 14]. Inflammation and scarring of lung parenchyma, the internal lung tissue, may also be caused by lung disease [13, 15]. Popular causes of such diseases include exposure to asbestos in the textile and shipping industries and exposure to silica in the sandblasting and concrete breaking industries [13, 16].

Industrialization has exposed workers to high levels of respiratory toxicants in developing countries, many of which have been successfully controlled in industrialized countries [13, 17, 18]. For example, a program to eradicate silicosis worldwide has been launched by the World Health Organization (WHO). Agricultural workers' respiratory health has also earned growing attention.

A number of narrative and systematic reviews, indicate that a substantial proportion of cases of COPD are indeed attributable to exposures in the workplace. Occupationally-related causes of COPD have been identified from a wide-range of industry based studies including those in: coal mining; work with crystalline silica in the construction industry, tunneling, brick manufacture, pottery and ceramic work, the silica sand industry and iron and steel foundry work; welding; cotton manufacture; and agriculture [16, 19]. Other occupations of concern are work in smelters, iron and steel processing, rubber and tyre manufacturing and exposure to wood dust, ceramic fibers and a range of chemicals such as cadmium, isocyanates, vanadium, polycyclic aromatic hydrocarbons, particularly in asphalt fumes, and those in spray painting, and in coke oven work [20, 21].

3.1 Occupational dust exposure and COPD

Productive dust refers to solid micro-particles produced by the activities of human production that can float for a long period of time in the production atmosphere. Industrial and agricultural development sectors, such as mining, machinery manufacturing, smelting, building materials, textiles, road construction, hydropower, and food industries, generate productive dust. It can be categorized as inorganic dust, organic dust, and mixed dust according to the composition of the dust. Mineral dust, metal dust, and artificial inorganic dust are inorganic dust; biological dust, plant dust, and animal dust are organic dust [22]. It is a significant hazardous occupational hazard that pollutes the workplace environment and affects workers' health, contributing to the creation of different occupational lung diseases. Studies stated that occupational dust exposure may be causally associated with the pathogenesis of COPD [23]. Different literature on coal miners' airflow obstruction concluded that there was an obvious link between exposure to coal dust and the creation of chronic obstruction of airflow. In-depth research on the role of occupational dust exposure in the occurrence and development of COPD is therefore of great importance in reducing its incidence and alleviating the burden of its disease [21, 24]. Based on prior observations and using new data from published literature, the association between occupational dust exposure and COPD risk was further evaluated [24].

3.2 Street sweepers and dust

In the maintaining of health and hygiene in cities, street sweepers play an important role. This work exposes street sweepers to a number of risk factors that make them vulnerable to some occupational diseases, such as dust, bioaerosols, volatile organic matter and mechanical stress (**Figure 2**). The major morbid conditions observed in these workers include respiratory and eye diseases, accidents, burns, cuts and wounds, skin infections, animal bites, etc. [25, 26].

Dusts are solid particles that, depending on their origin, physical characteristics and environmental conditions, may be or become airborne, varying in size from below 1 μm to at least 100 μm [27].

Examples of the dust types contained in the working environment include:

- Mineral dust, such as free crystalline silica (e.g. quartz), coal and cement dust;
- Metallic particles, such as dust of lead, cadmium, nickel, and beryllium;
- Other chemical dusts, e.g., many bulk chemicals and pesticides:
- Dusts of organic and vegetables, such as flour, wood, cotton and tea dusts, pollen;
- Biohazards, such as viable particles, spores and molds

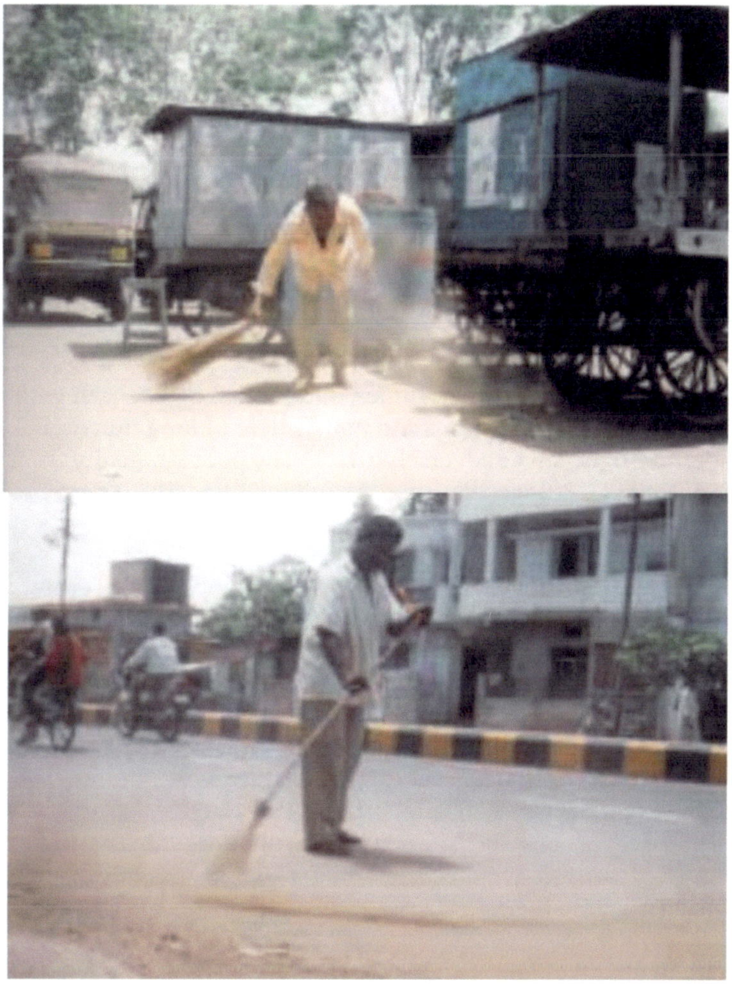

Figure 2.
Street sweeper at work, not using any protective devices [25].

In the gaseous phase (gases and vapors) or as aerosols, airborne pollutants exist. In the form of airborne particles, sprays, mist, smoke and fumes, aerosols can exist. Both these types may be relevant in the occupational setting since they contribute to a wide range of occupational diseases. Airborne dust is of particular concern since it is well known that it is associated with typical widespread occupational pulmonary diseases such as pneumoconiosis, as well as systemic intoxications such as lead poisoning, especially at higher exposure levels. Other dust-related illnesses, such as cancer, asthma, allergic alveolitis and irritation, as well as a wide variety of non-respiratory diseases, which can occur at much lower levels of exposure, are also increasingly involved in the modern period.

3.3 Penetration and deposition mechanism of dust particles in human respiratory regions

Dust particles small enough to stay airborne may be inhaled through the nasal route (nose) or the oral route. Dust passes through the different regions of nasopharyngeal or extra-thoracic region, trachea-bronchial region and alveolar region. The probability of inhalation depends on particle aerodynamic diameter, air movement around the body and breathing rate. The inhaled particles may then either be deposited or exhaled again, depending on a whole range of physiological and particle-related factors.

Tiny dust particles have the potential to penetrate the lungs and the body more easily posing a risk to the health of exposed individuals. Although coarse dust is collected in the airways that conduct (nasal passages and bronchi). The fine dust in the bronchioles will enter (smaller airways). Ultrafine dust is almost entirely capable of accessing the deepest regions of the lungs (the alveoli) where oxygen reaches the blood and waste gases are left to be exhaled.

3.4 Effects of dust on the respiratory function

Occupational exposures to dust, fumes, and gases are associated with increased prevalence of respiratory symptoms and impairment of lung function. Any part of the respiratory tract can be adversely affected by poor air quality from the nose to the alveoli [23, 28] mechanisms, the inherent toxicity of particles, pattern of deposition, removal from the respiratory tract and the properties of the air contaminants (WHO, 2005).

The respiratory problems caused by dust exposure include chest pain, occasional cough, occasional shortness of breath and wheezing. Dust inhalation over time contributes to proliferation and fibrotic changes in the lungs. Severity depends on many factors, including the chemical nature, physical condition of the material inhaled, size, dust particle concentration, length of exposure, and individual susceptibility to exposure. The extent of impact is influenced by the proximity to sensitive receptors, wind speed, velocity and nature of work topography. The reaction of the respiratory system to inhaled particles largely depends on where the particles settle. The most important lung reactions occur in the deepest regions of the lungs. Dust particles and dust containing macrophages collect in the lung tissues, causing injury to the lungs [28].

3.5 Exposure to disinfectants with incidence of chronic obstructive pulmonary disease

Exposure to cleaning products and disinfectants is prevalent at work and at home, and among women it is more common. In the health care sector, exposure levels are particularly high. There is a growing awareness of the respiratory health risks associated with exposure to cleaning products and disinfectants. Studying a wider variety of respiratory effects confirms the irritant properties of certain chemicals used in disinfectants. Studies have documented an increased risk of COPD among cleaning workers, an accelerated decrease in lung function and higher rates of death due to COPD.

3.5.1 Cleaning agents

A cleaning product is defined as any material used in general work environments to clean or disinfect surfaces. These items have become an essential part of everyday life, as they are used in almost all workplaces and homes on a daily basis. To facilitate dust and dirt removal, and for disinfection and surface maintenance, a wide range of cleaning agents have been developed [29]. In general, cleaning agents can be defined as natural or synthetic substances used to assist with the cleaning process.

However, cleaning is not without risks. Both volatile and non-volatile compounds contain cleaning agents. Excessive exposure to potentially harmful volatile contaminants results from the application of popular cleaning products [29].

For staff, cleaning materials have emerged as a major respiratory threat. Most cleaning agents (e.g. chlorine and ammonia) have an irritating effect on mucous membranes and the skin and have a sensitizing ability (e.g. monoethanolamine and aldehydes). These products have also been implicated in numerous respiratory disorders, including job-related asthma [29, 30].

The glass cleaner and other hard-surface cleaner chemicals also contain ammonia, which can irritate the skin, eyes, mouth, and lungs. A family of chemicals recognized for their disinfectant and detergent properties are ammonium quaternary compounds. They are found in cleaning products such as disinfectant sprays and toilet cleaners, and have been identified among cleaning workers as a known cause of occupational asthma [31, 32].

The most widely used disinfecting and cleaning agent is chlorine bleach or sodium hypochlorite. It is also used for various applications in everyday life, such as water and food disinfection and surface cleaning in public and private buildings [33]. Chlorine bleach, however, is unstable and is a highly reactive chemical. Chlorine bleach can emit chlorine or tri-chloramine, two gases that are significant irritants to the eyes and the respiratory tract, when mixed with other cleaning agents. Chlorine gas exposure can lead to coughing, shortness of breath, chest pain, nausea, and other symptoms [31, 33]. The acute inhalation of respiratory irritants such as hypochlorite and chlorine gas at toxic concentrations results in a clinical entity known as reactive airway dysfunction syndrome [34].

Monoethanolamine (MEA) is a surfactant that is frequently found in detergents that improves its cleaning efficiency. MEA is used in cleaning items such as laundry detergents and floor cleaners and has been described as a suspected occupational asthma inducer for cleaning employees [31].

Aldehydes are commonly used to clean heat-sensitive devices, such as fiber optic endoscopes, in medical facilities. They may induce hypersensitivity reactions induced by mucous irritation, respiratory symptoms and immunoglobulin IgE, and are well-known causative agents of occupational asthma [29].

4. COPD and its effect on work

The burden of chronic obstructive pulmonary disease (COPD) and its effect on quality of life is well known. Of the main long-term health conditions, there is a growing interest in the impact of chronic obstructive pulmonary disease (COPD) on the ability to work [35, 36]. As COPD progresses patients are increasingly faced with a number of functional limitations, and as a result, can experience effects on their personal, social and work life [36, 37].

COPD is a debilitating disease affecting the daily lives of patients. Having COPD adversely affects patients' rates of employment and work productivity. Physical activity levels are low even in patients in the early stages of COPD [38]. Increasing severity of COPD is associated with decreasing physical activity [39]. In a more recent study of approximately 2,500 patients aged 45–67 years in Brazil, China, Germany, Turkey, the United States, and the United Kingdom, nearly 40% retired early due to COPD at an average age of 54 years, and several subsequent studies have shown that people with COPD are more likely not working because of COPD. In certain cases, failure to work can indicate the fact that occupational exposure worsens symptoms and, of course, exposure may also lead to the development of COPD (**Figure 3**). COPD employees indicated that problems causing them to stop working involved work that worsening their COPD [40, 41].

In addition to causing work to stop, COPD contributes to increased absenteeism. People with COPD are almost half as likely to have a short-term disability and are

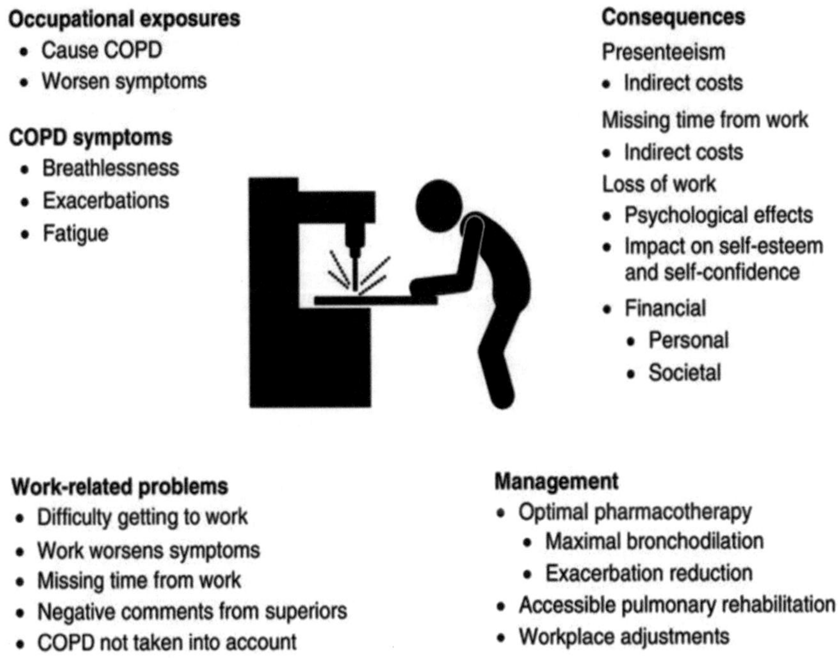

Figure 3.
Chronic obstructive pulmonary disease (COPD) and work [40].

more than four times more likely to have a long-term disability, but this can also be affected by comorbidity. The efficacy of patients who stay at work can also be limited by symptoms (**Figure 3**). In the United States and other nations, a number of major cross-sectional studies showed that people with COPD were substantially more likely to report presentism, and findings from studies using self-report data suggest that about 13–18 percent are restricted in what they can do [40].

Working generally has a positive effect on health and functioning [40]. There is increasing evidence that being in work is good for physical and mental health and wellbeing. Being in work provides a feeling of self-worth but also has economic advantages for both the individual and society. Evidence suggests that being out of work may be harmful for individuals [4].

Becoming unemployed, together with lower self-esteem and trust, is associated with significantly higher levels of depression and anxiety; however, it can lead to improved physical health in the short term, particularly when symptoms have been aggravated by working conditions. In countries that do not have welfare programs to help the unemployed or in which healthcare must be paid for, the impact of COPD-related loss of jobs on individuals is likely to be highest [42]. In 2010, 384 million people are projected to have COPD worldwide, with the largest burden falling in Latin America, Sub-Saharan Africa, India, China, and Southeast Asia. Compared to average earnings, the cost of medicine is very high in many of these countries, and its availability across government health services is low. These costs intensify the financial insecurity of households in low- and middle-income countries without an income and may push patients to fund treatment by household borrowing and selling functional properties [40].

Occupational chronic respiratory diseases pose a public health concern with economic consequences in all countries. In the world's poorest countries, innovations which are outdated or banned in developed countries are still largely used. Occupational diseases are usually less apparent and are not sufficiently regarded as an issue in low and middle income countries. In addition, most patients are not paid in those countries and typically continue to function until the illness is serious and disabling.

5. Conclusion

Chronic obstructive pulmonary disease (COPD) is a slowly progressive, potentially highly disabling, respiratory condition with many potential causes. COPD is a major cause of chronic morbidity and mortality throughout the world. Many people suffer from this disease for years and die prematurely from it or its complications. The most important risk factor of developing COPD is cigarette smoking; however, occupational exposure, exposure to air pollutions, and respiratory infections can also be attributed to developing COPD. Workers in various occupations such as mining, construction, and even office buildings are exposed to respiratory toxicants, which can cause disease at any point along the respiratory tract. The dusts from coal, stone quarries, wood, cereals and agricultural work, animal stables, textiles, and paper production that can arise in occupational environments have been regulated by the International Labor Organization and considered possible as contributors to COPD. A better understanding of these causes paves the way for effective interventions to reduce the future incidence of this unpleasant condition. There is a growing interest in the impact of chronic obstructive pulmonary disease on the ability to work. As COPD progresses patients are increasingly faced with a number of functional limitations, and as a result, can experience effects on their personal, social and work life.

Conflict of interest

The authors declare that they have no competing interest.

Author details

Biruk Getahun[1]* and Abebe Ayalew Bekel[2]

1 Department of Medical Physiology, School of Medicine, College of Medicine and Health Sciences, Bahir Dar University, Bahir Dar, Ethiopia

2 Department of Human Anatomy, School of Medicine, College of Medicine and Health Sciences, Bahir Dar University, Bahir Dar, Ethiopia

*Address all correspondence to: birukkgetahun@gmail.com

References

[1] Trupin L, Earnest G, San Pedro M, Balmes JR, Eisner MD, Yelin E, Katz PP, Blanc PD. The occupational burden of chronic obstructive pulmonary disease. European Respiratory Journal. 2003; 22(3):462-9.

[2] Cho Y, Lee J, Choi M, Choi W, Myong JP, Kim HR, Koo JW. Work-related COPD after years of occupational exposure. Annals of occupational and environmental medicine. 2015; 27(1).

[3] Naidoo R. Work-related chronic obstructive pulmonary disease. Continuing Medical Education. 2009; 27(11).

[4] Kalirai KK. The effects of Chronic Obstructive Pulmonary Disease on work related outcomes (Doctoral dissertation, University of Birmingham); 2016.

[5] Levy ML, Quanjer PH, Rachel B, Cooper BG, Holmes S, Small IR. Diagnostic Spirometry in Primary Care: Proposed standards for general practice compliant with American Thoracic Society and European Respiratory Society recommendations. Primary Care Respiratory Journal. 2009; 18(3):130-47.

[6] West JB. Respiratory physiology: the essentials. Lippincott Williams & Wilkins; 2012.

[7] Eisner MD, Anthonisen N, Coultas D, Kuenzli N, Perez-Padilla R, Postma D, Romieu I, Silverman EK, Balmes JR. An official American Thoracic Society public policy statement: Novel risk factors and the global burden of chronic obstructive pulmonary disease. American journal of respiratory and critical care medicine. 2010; 182(5):693-718.

[8] Williamson JP, Twaddell SH, Lee YG, Salamonsen M, Hew M, Fielding D, Nguyen P, Steinfort D, Hopkins P, Smith N, Grainge C. Thoracic ultrasound recognition of competence: a position paper of the Thoracic Society of Australia and New Zealand. Respirology. 2017; 22(2):405-8.

[9] Torén K, Vikgren J, Olin AC, Rosengren A, Bergström G, Brandberg J. Occupational exposure to vapor, gas, dust, or fumes and chronic airflow limitation, COPD, and emphysema: the Swedish CArdioPulmonary BioImage Study (SCAPIS pilot). International journal of chronic obstructive pulmonary disease. 2017; 12:3407.

[10] Sadhra S, Kurmi OP, Sadhra SS, Lam KB, Ayres JG. Occupational COPD and job exposure matrices: a systematic review and meta-analysis. International journal of chronic obstructive pulmonary disease. 2017; 12:725.

[11] Mazitova NN, Saveliev AA, Berheeva ZM, Amirov NK. COPD and occupation: a retrospective cohort study of industrial workers. Archives of Industrial Hygiene and Toxicology. 2012; 63(3):345-56.

[12] Balmes J, Becklake M, Blanc P, Henneberger P. American Thoracic Society Statement: Occupational contribution to the burden of airway disease. American journal of respiratory and critical care medicine. 2003; 167(5):787.

[13] Lemière C, Vandenplas O. Occupational Allergy. InMiddleton's Allergy Essentials 2017; (pp. 361-375). Elsevier.

[14] GBD 2016 Occupational Chronic Respiratory Risk Factors Collaborators. Global and regional burden of chronic respiratory disease in 2016 arising from non-infectious airborne occupational exposures: a systematic analysis for the Global Burden of Disease Study

2016. Occupational and environmental medicine. 2020; 77(3):142-50.

[15] De Matteis S, Heederik D, Burdorf A, Colosio C, Cullinan P, Henneberger PK, Olsson A, Raynal A, Rooijackers J, Santonen T, Sastre J. Current and new challenges in occupational lung diseases. European Respiratory Review. 2017; 26(146).

[16] Hnizdo E, Vallyathan V. Chronic obstructive pulmonary disease due to occupational exposure to silica dust: a review of epidemiological and pathological evidence. Occupational and environmental medicine. 2003; 60(4):237-43.

[17] Torén K, Järvholm B. Effect of occupational exposure to vapors, gases, dusts, and fumes on COPD mortality risk among Swedish construction workers: a longitudinal cohort study. Chest. 2014; 145(5):992-7.

[18] Maio S, Baldacci S, Carrozzi L, Pistelli F, Viegi G. The global burden of chronic respiratory diseases. Breathe. 2006; 3(1):20-9.

[19] Rushton L. Chronic obstructive pulmonary disease and occupational exposure to silica. Reviews on environmental health. 2007; 22(4):255-72.

[20] Dodd KE, Mazurek JM. Prevalence of COPD among workers with work-related asthma. Journal of Asthma. 2020; 57(11):1179-87.

[21] Rosenberg SR, Kalhan R, Mannino DM. Epidemiology of chronic obstructive pulmonary disease: prevalence, morbidity, mortality, and risk factors. InSeminars in respiratory and critical care medicine 2015; 36(4): 457-469.

[22] Fishwick D, Sen D, Barber C, Bradshaw L, Robinson E, Sumner J, COPD Standard Collaboration Group. Occupational chronic obstructive pulmonary disease: a standard of care. Occupational Medicine. 2015; 65(4):270-82.

[23] Peng C, Yan Y, Li Z, Jiang Y, Cai Y. Chronic obstructive pulmonary disease caused by inhalation of dust: A meta-analysis. Medicine. 2020; 99(34).

[24] Oxman AD, Muir DC, Shannon HS, Stock SR, Hnizdo E, Lange HJ. Occupational dust exposure and chronic obstructive pulmonary disease: a systematic overview of the evidence. American Review of Respiratory Disease. 2012.

[25] Sabde YD, Zodpey SP. A study of morbidity pattern in street sweepers: a cross-sectional study. Indian Journal of Community Medicine: Official Publication of Indian Association of Preventive & Social Medicine. 2008; 33(4):224.

[26] Dalju I, Dessie A, Bogale L, Mekonnen TH. Occupational risk factors associated with respiratory symptoms among tannery workers in Mojo town, Southeast Ethiopia, 2018: a comparative cross-sectional study. Multidisciplinary Respiratory Medicine. 2019; 14(1):27.

[27] World Health Organization. The world health report, (2002); pp.81-92.

[28] World Health Organization (WHO). Hazard prevention and control in the work environment: airborne dust. 2005.

[29] Quirce, S. & Barranco, P. (2010). Cleaning agents and asthma. J Investig Allergol Clin Immunol, 20, 542-50.

[30] Dumas O, Varraso R, Boggs KM, Quinot C, Zock JP, Henneberger PK, Speizer FE, Le Moual N, Camargo CA. Association of occupational exposure to disinfectants with incidence of chronic obstructive pulmonary disease among US female nurses. JAMA network open. 2019; 2(10):e1913563.

[31] Gorman A. Household hazards: Potential hazards of home cleaning products. Women's Voices for the Earth; 2007.

[32] Driscoll T, Steenland K, Nelson DI, Leigh J, Prüss-Üstün A, Campbell-Lendrum DH, Corvalán CF, Woodward A, World Health Organization. Occupational airborne particulates: Assessing the environmental burden of disease at national and local levels. World Health Organization; 2004.

[33] Nickmilder M, Carbonnelle S, Bernard A. House cleaning with chlorine bleach and the risks of allergic and respiratory diseases in children. Pediatric allergy and immunology. 2007; 18(1):27-35.

[34] DEMİRALAY R. Effects of the use of hypochlorite as a cleaning substance on pulmonary functions. Turkish Journal of Medical Sciences. 2001; 31(1):51-7.

[35] Rai KK, Adab P, Ayres JG, Jordan RE. Systematic review: chronic obstructive pulmonary disease and work-related outcomes. Occupational Medicine. 2018; 68(2):99-108.

[36] de Sousa Sena R, Ahmed S, Tan WC, Li PZ, Labonté L, Aaron SD, Benedetti A, Chapman KR, Walker B, Fitzgerald JM, Hernandez P. Work productivity loss in mild to moderate COPD: lessons learned from the CanCOLD study. European Respiratory Journal. 2017; 50(3).

[37] Fishwick D, Barber CM, Darby AC. Review series: Occupational and environmental lung disease: Chronic obstructive pulmonary disease and the workplace. Chronic Respiratory Disease. 2010; 7(2):113-22.

[38] Onoue A, Omori H, Katoh T, Kubota K, Nonami Y, Ogata Y, Inoue H. Relationship of airflow limitation severity with work productivity reduction and sick leave in a Japanese working population. International journal of chronic obstructive pulmonary disease. 2016; 11:567.

[39] Bepko J, Mansalis K. Common occupational disorders: asthma, COPD, dermatitis, and musculoskeletal disorders. American family physician. 2016; 93(12):1000-6.

[40] Halpin D. Chronic Obstructive Pulmonary Disease and Work: Is It Time to Stop? Am J Respir Crit Care Med. 2019; 200(10): 1195-1207.

[41] Fan Y, Xu W, Wang Y, Wang Y, Yu S, Ye Q. Association of occupational dust exposure with combined chronic obstructive pulmonary disease and pneumoconiosis: a cross-sectional study in China. BMJ open. 2020; 10(9):e038874.

[42] Sin DD, Stafinski T, Ng YC, Bell NR, Jacobs P. The impact of chronic obstructive pulmonary disease on work loss in the United States. American journal of respiratory and critical care medicine. 2002; 165(5):704-7.

Chapter 4

COPD-Related Factors Affect the Quality of Life of Patients

Maha Dardouri and Manel Mallouli

Abstract

Over the past decades, health-related quality of life (HRQL) has become a major topic of research in the context of chronic conditions, including chronic obstructive pulmonary disease (COPD). HRQL assessment became a part of the mandatory criteria for judging the effectiveness of a therapeutic care plan. COPD still imposes an enormous burden on patients and health care systems. Daily symptoms, poor pulmonary function, and medication use can affect the social and physical life components of patients. Indeed, HRQL predictors in COPD patients were controversial in the literature. To this end, we conducted a review of the literature to describe COPD-related factors that influence the HRQL of patients. This study included research articles published in English from 2010 to 2020. This review of sparse and well-designed literature gave a current state-of-the-art that could be useful for clinicians, and in establishing advanced COPD management plans.

Keywords: COPD, quality of life, dyspnea, exacerbation, comorbidity, disease management

1. Introduction

Chronic obstructive pulmonary disease (COPD) is a lung disease that is characterized by a persistent blockage of the flow of inhaled gases. It tends to be an under-diagnosed condition, which engages the life prognosis [1]. In fact, COPD is a growing global health problem that caused 4.07% of total disability adjusted life years in adults aged 50 to 69 years [2]. It is currently the fourth leading cause of death worldwide [3]. More than 3 million people worldwide died of COPD in 2012, which was equal to 6% of all deaths globally [4].

Although this condition is not curable, pharmacological and non-pharmacological treatments can slow the progression of the disease [1]. Symptoms, such as dyspnea, cough, and sputum, can lead to exercise intolerance and restriction in daily life activities of patients with COPD [5, 6]. Consequently, they progressively impair the health related quality of life (HRQL) [6]. According to Roche and Similowski, impaired HRQL is a major issue in chronic disease management. Its measurement is currently part of the mandatory criteria for judging the effectiveness of a treatment or a plan of chronic condition management [7].

Indeed, HRQL was defined by the World Health Organization since 1984 as the individual's perception of his place in life, in the context of the culture and value system in which he or she lives, in relation to his objectives, expectations, standards and concerns. It is a very broad concept, influenced in a complex way by the physical health of the person, his or her psychological state, his or her level of independence, his or her social relations, as well as his or her relationship to the essential elements of his or her environment [8]. This perception may vary with age, health status, maturity, and over time [9, 10]. Thus, it is important to periodically assess the HRQL of patients.

In fact, HRQL assessment is an important indicator in healthcare since it provides an overview of the impact of the disease on the patient's life. It is substantial for optimizing patient comfort and improving care [7]. In research, HRQL assessment is interesting to justify various forms of treatment. It helps in improving therapies and providing significant data to judge the Cost/Effectiveness ratio of healthcare therapies [11].

One of the main objectives of COPD treatment was to improve the general health condition of patients. As a result, HRQL has become a major topic of research in COPD patients [12, 13]. Several studies assessed the factors determining the HRQL in patients with COPD using various methods and instruments. Indeed, predictors of HRQL were controversial in the literature. Furthermore, it is crucial to identify clinical factors related to COPD that affect the HRQL of patients. This could be useful and time-saving for health care providers in developing advanced and evidence-based COPD management programs.

In this chapter, we aimed to describe the findings of studies that analyzed clinical factors determining the HRQL of COPD patients published in the past decade.

2. Methods

2.1 Study design

This was a literature review of analytical studies that assessed the clinical factors determining the HRQL in patients with COPD.

2.2 Sources of information and data search

The data search was carried out using three electronic databases, namely, MEDLINE, ScienceDirect, and Mendeley. Data collection was conducted from December 2020 to January 2021. Studies identified in the references of the selected articles, and that met the inclusion criteria were included in this review.

The terms used for the search were 'quality of life', 'Pulmonary Disease, Chronic Obstructive', 'epidemiologic factors', 'risk factors', 'influencing factors', 'outcomes and process assessment' in different combinations.

2.3 Inclusion criteria

Studies were primarily assessed basing on their titles and abstracts. After exclusion of duplicates, studies were included in this review according to the following inclusion criteria: English language articles published in scientific journals, the study included generic or specific instruments or both of them to collect information on predictors of HRQL among COPD patients, the study included only COPD patients, the work included quantitative information on clinical predictors of HRQL and articles published from 2010 to 2020.

2.4 Data extraction

For each study included in this literature review, the following variables were recorded: author and country, study design, study period, sample size, tools for HRQL assessment, and findings of the study regarding clinical factors influencing HRQL.

3. Results

Basing on the titles and abstracts, forty-two articles seemed to meet the objectives of this review. Twenty-six articles were excluded for one of the following reasons: articles not written in English language, articles published before 2010 (n = 24), samples were not exclusively COPD patients, articles aimed to assess HRQL without identifying predictive factors. Consequently, the final sample was reduced to sixteen studies.

Table 1 shows the characteristics of the included studies. The studies were conducted in different regions in the world, namely European countries, South Korea, China, Egypt, Tunisia, and United States. Most of the studies used a multicenter, cross-sectional analytical design, with studies' periods ranged from 3 months to 6 years. Five studies used a multicenter, prospective analytical design, with 6-month to 5-year period [14–18]. The minimal sample size used in the studies was n = 42, and the maximum one was 5619. The mean age of studied populations ranged from 59 ± 10.1 to 72.2 ± 8.11. Patients with all COPD severity stages (GOLD I to IV) and with co-morbidities were included in the studies.

Various tools of HRQL assessment were used in the literature (**Table 1**). The St George's Respiratory Questionnaire (SGRQ), which is a COPD-specific tool, was largely used (10 studies). Two studies used the COPD Assessment Test [19, 20].

Regarding generic instruments, the Medical Outcome Study 36-Item Short-Form Health Survey (SF-36) and the EuroQol-5 Dimension (EQ-5D) were used in 6 studies. Also the Medical Outcome Study 12-Item Short-Form Health Survey (SF-12) was used in one study as a second tool. The severity of dyspnea was mainly assessed by the "Medical Research Council (MRC) dyspnea scale".

All of the studies reported a significant HRQL impairment in patients with COPD. The prospective studies recorded the changes of HRQL status over time at 6 months to 5 years' follow-up.

Twelve papers identified more than one clinical factor affecting the HRQL in COPD subjects, and five articles identified only one factor [18, 19, 21–23]. COPD symptoms [14–16, 18, 21, 23–26], COPD severity [5, 6, 12, 24, 27], and co-morbidities [5, 12, 16, 20, 24, 26, 27] were commonly identified as predictors of HRQL in COPD subjects.

4. Discussion

The current review reported sixteen studies with two different designs: cross sectional and prospective. The cross sectional study design is limited in its ability to draw valid conclusions as to the association between COPD-related factors and HRQL. Also, cross-sectional studies can present a memorization bias. Nevertheless, the sample size used in most of the documented studies was large enough to assess HRQL with adequate precision. In regards with prospective studies (n = 5), they eliminate the memorization bias as there is no need for information recall. Follow-up can provide more information concerning the changes that patients experience and their possible impact on HRQL. For instance, Monteagudo and colleagues observed a clinically important changes in HRQL in nearly two thirds of the study population (36.7% improving and 29.2% worsening HRQL). However, the loss to follow-up is common in prospective studies, which is an important limitation [28].

Author(s), year, country of the study	n	Study period	Study design	HRQL Instrument(s)	Clinical factors predicting HRQL of patients with COPD
Jones et al. (2011), Europe	1817	5 months	Cross-sectional epidemiological, non-randomized study.	St George's Respiratory Questionnaire, Short Form 12.	Severity of COPD, exacerbation, presence of three or more co-morbidities.
Zamzam et al. (2012), Egypt	40	1 year	Cross-sectional study	St George's Respiratory Questionnaire.	Severity of COPD, Smoking index, forced expiratory volume in 1 second (FEV1), FEV1/FVC ratio (FVC: Forced vital capacity), Peak expiratory flow rate (PEFR), Forced expiratory flow at 25%- 75% of maximal lung volume (FEF25–75%).
Monteagudo et al. (2013), Spain	791	1 year	Multi center, prospective study	St George's Respiratory Questionnaire.	Factors associated with HRQL improvement: Poly-medication, pulmonology visits, and a balanced diet; ending respiratory rehabilitation, quitting smoking habit, infrequent exacerbation. Factors associated with HRQL worsening: Symptoms (dyspnea, expectoration), hospital admissions
Negi et el (2014), India	126	6 months	Cross-sectional study	St George's Respiratory Questionnaire.	Severity of COPD, body mass index, FEV1, dyspnea, depression, anxiety, smoking index.
Liang et al. (2014), China	491	1 year	Prospective cohort study	St George's Respiratory Questionnaire.	MRC dyspnea grade, number of exacerbations
Sundh et al. (2015), Sweden	373	11 months	Multicenter, cross-sectional study	EuroQol-5 dimension, COPD Assessment Test.	Co-morbid conditions: chronic bronchitis, depression, osteoporosis, and musculoskeletal symptoms
Kendrovà et al. (2015), Slovakia	80	7 months	Cross-sectional study	St George's Respiratory Questionnaire, Short Form-36	Symptoms: cough, dyspnea
Deslee et al. (2016), France	178	—	Cross-sectional multicenter study	St George's Respiratory Questionnaire.	Current cough in the previous 7 days.

Author(s), year, country of the study	n	Study period	Study design	HRQL Instrument(s)	Clinical factors predicting HRQL of patients with COPD
Martinez et al. (2016), United States	5619	—	Cross-sectional study	St George's Respiratory Questionnaire.	Dyspnea severity.
Kwon & Kim (2016), South Korea	2,734	6-year data	Cross-sectional surveys	EuroQol-5 dimension	Severity of COPD, co-morbidities (Depression, osteoporosis, diabetes, cardiovascular disease)
Lee et al. (2017), South Korea	1,264	4 years	Multi center, prospective study	St George's Respiratory Questionnaire.	Symptoms (dyspnea and cough), number of co-morbidities.
Mallouli et al. (2017), Tunisia	335	3 months	Cross-sectional study	Medical Outcome Study 36-Item Short-Form Health Survey (MOS SF-36)	COPD severity (Moderate to very severe), 2 or more co-morbidities, MRC dyspnea grade 4 and 5.
Brien et al. (2018), United Kingdom	735	2 years	Cross-sectional study	5 level EuroQol-5 dimension (EQ-5D 5 L)	Dyspnea, depression, anxiety, 12-month exacerbations.
Amini et al. (2020), Iran	175	11 months	Cross-sectional study	Chronic Obstructive Pulmonary Disease Assessment Test	Inhaler technique
Esteban et al. (2020), Spain	543	5 years	Prospective cohort study	St George's Respiratory Questionnaire.	Inhaled medication, smoking habit, FEV1, 6MWT distance, body mass index, residual volume, diffusing capacity of the lung for carbon monoxide, physical activity, and hospitalization.
Park (2020), South Korea	42	6 months	Longitudinal study	Medical Outcome Study 36-Item Short-Form Health Survey (MOS SF-36)	COPD symptoms

Table 1.
Characteristics of the Studies analyzing clinical outcomes influencing the HRQL of patients with COPD.

Regarding to the populations' characteristics, most of the studies addressed middle-age adults and/or older adults. Besides, most of the patients were between moderate and very severe COPD severity stages. They presented different comorbidities, such as diabetes, osteoporosis, depression, anxiety, and cardiovascular diseases.

HRQL is a multidimensional, subjective, and dynamic concept, which make it difficult to assess. Nevertheless, there are reliable and valid HRQL measurement tools in the literature. Indeed, Mercier and Schraub distinguished two methods to assess HRQL [29]. The first one is via psychological interview that allows a comprehensive evaluation of HRQL and has therapeutic value. The second method is via psychometric tools that consist of scales or questionnaires. It performs a restrictive evaluation of HRQL and allows standardized measurement. This method is generally easy to use. For that, we included the studies that used this type of HRQL evaluation in this review.

In the literature, the specific questionnaire mostly used to assess the HRQL was the St George's Respiratory Questionnaire. The generic questionnaires SF-36 and the EQ-5D were also widely used in the literature. These instruments reported that COPD altered the HRQL of patients even in a mild stage [5, 6, 14, 15, 21, 23–25].

HRQL is the result of the interaction of multiple physical, psychological and social components. Consequently, several factors can affect it, especially in COPD subjects.

This review demonstrated that multiple COPD-related factors had a significant negative influence on the HRQL of patients with COPD.

4.1 COPD-related factors

COPD-related factors include pulmonary function, physical activity, chronic cough, chronic wheeze, dyspnea, exacerbations, and hospitalizations. The first concept related to a chronic disease is the severity stage. Therefore, the impact of COPD severity on HRQL was often analyzed. Five studies demonstrated that HRQL was deteriorated across severity stages of COPD [5, 6, 12, 24, 27]. Indeed, the more the disease worsens the more the HRQL deteriorates. Thus, it is important to note that HRQL should be considered as a substantial health status indicator in this population.

Symptoms, including chronic cough/sputum, wheeze, and dyspnea, were commonly identified as predictors of HRQL (9 studies). Eight of nine studies showed that an advanced dyspnea grade was associated with a worsening of HRQL scores [14–16, 21, 23–26]. Frequent cough [21, 22] and expectoration [14] also deteriorated the HRQL scores.

The negative impact of exacerbations was reported in the literature. Authors declared that the degree of HRQL impairment depended on the frequency of exacerbations [5, 14, 15]. Indeed, Liang and colleagues revealed that COPD patients who had 3 exacerbations or more in the past 1 year had significantly an impaired HRQL [15].

One the main objectives of COPD treatment was to improve the patient's health status. Indeed, Monteagudo and colleagues revealed that patients taking multiple medications and ending respiratory rehabilitation had improved HRQL at 1-year follow-up [14]. Recently, Esteban and colleagues showed that using 2 out of long-acting beta agonists, long-acting muscarinic antagonists, and inhaled corticosteroid, or 3 of them was significantly associated with HRQL scores [17]. Amini and colleagues demonstrated that appropriate inhaler technique was associated with better HRQL in patients with COPD [19]. This data suggested that optimizing inhaler technique should be considered in COPD management programs.

Pulmonary function was significantly associated with HRQL [6, 17, 24]. It was shown that residual volume, diffusing capacity of the lung for carbon monoxide, and low forced expiratory volume in 1 second (FEV1) predicted HRQL of COPD patients.

In brief, dyspnea had significantly and independently the highest impact on HRQL in comparison with other COPD- related factors and co-morbidities [12, 14–16, 24, 26]. Several research studies demonstrated that dyspnea was the best predictor of HRQL in COPD patients, especially MRC dyspnea grade 4 and 5 [15, 16, 26]. Indeed, Monteagudo and colleagues revealed that the onset of new symptoms negatively influenced HRQL more than their persistence [14].

4.2 Co-morbidities

Patients with COPD often have at least one associated co-morbidity. Co-morbidities were significantly associated with HRQL impairment. Studies showed that the degree of impairment depended on the number of co-morbidities [5, 12, 16]. Indeed, COPD patients who had 2 to 3 or more co-morbidities had significantly lower HRQL score. Anxiety, depression and other chronic diseases, such as diabetes, hypertension, osteoporosis, and cardiovascular disease, were associated with HRQL impairment [20, 24, 26, 27]. In fact, several studies showed that depression was commonly associated with HRQL worsening [20, 24, 26, 27]. Brien and colleagues reported that depression was associated with higher HRQL [26]. Besides, Kwon and Kim showed that osteoporosis and depression had the highest impact on HRQL in comparison with cardiovascular disease, diabetes, cancer and hypertension [27]. However, Sundh and colleagues revealed that chronic bronchitis phenotype in COPD patients indicated a higher risk of low HRQL in comparison with musculoskeletal symptoms, osteoporosis and depression [20].

Coping strategies can enhance the HRQL of COPD patients, but this might fail in case of co-morbid conditions [30]. Therefore, COPD management interventions should address co-morbid conditions along with COPD-related factors. Patient-tailored care could be an appropriate strategy for optimal management of the disease and its associated factors.

5. Conclusions

To conclude, COPD is a burdensome disease that progressively deteriorates the HRQL of patients. This literature review reported that disease severity, frequent symptoms and exacerbations, poor lung function, inappropriate medication use and co-morbidities were significantly associated with HRQL impairment. Dyspnea had the highest impact on HRQL in comparison with other COPD-related factors. Besides, depression was commonly associated with a higher impairment of HRQL. These factors should no longer be a matter of controversy. Disease management interventions should be delivered as early as possible in order to prevent the onset of new co-morbidities and to optimize the disease control.

Acknowledgements

The authors declare that this work was not funded.

Conflict of interest

The authors declare no conflict of interest.

Author details

Maha Dardouri[1,2*] and Manel Mallouli[3]

1 Higher School of Health Sciences and Techniques, University of Sousse, Sousse, Tunisia

2 Research Laboratory LR12ES03 "Quality of Care and Management of Maternal HEALTH Services", Faculty of Medicine of Sousse, University of Sousse, Sousse, Tunisia

3 Research Laboratory LR12ES03 "Quality of Care and Management of Maternal Health Services", Department of Community and Family Medicine, Faculty of Medicine, University of Sousse, Sousse, Tunisia

*Address all correspondence to: maha.dardouri@famso.u-sousse.tn

References

[1] World Health Organization. Chronic obstructive pulmonary disease (COPD), https://www.who.int/news-room/fact-sheets/detail/chronic-obstructive-pulmonary-disease-(copd) (2017, accessed 16 February 2021).

[2] Institute for Health Metrics and Evaluation. Global Burden Disease Compare, https://vizhub.healthdata.org/gbd-compare/ (2019, accessed 8 February 2021).

[3] Lozano R, Naghavi M, Foreman K, et al. Global and regional mortality from 235 causes of death for 20 age groups in 1990 and 2010: A systematic analysis for the Global Burden of Disease Study 2010. *Lancet* 2012; 380: 2095-2128.

[4] Global Initiative for Chronic Obstructive Lung Disease. GOLD Report 2020. Glob Initiat Chronic Obstr Lung Dis 2020; 141.

[5] Jones PW, Brusselle G, Dal Negro RW, et al. Health-related quality of life in patients by COPD severity within primary care in Europe. Respir Med 2011; 105: 57-66.

[6] Zamzam M, Azaba N, El Wahsha R, et al. Quality of life in COPD patients. Egypt J Chest Dis Tuberc 2012; 61: 281-289.

[7] Roche N, Similowski T. *Qualité de vie et BPCO*. John Libbey Eurotext, https://livre.fnac.com/a1916725/ROCHE-N-SIMILOWSKI-T-Qualite-de-vie-et-BPCO (2007, accessed 16 February 2021).

[8] World Health Organization. *Health promotion : a discussion document on the concept and principles : summary report of the Working Group on Concept and Principles of Health Promotion*, https://apps.who.int/iris/handle/10665/107835 (1984, accessed 16 February 2021).

[9] Debout C. Quality of life implications in the discipline of nursing. Soins Rev Réf Infirm 2004; 682 Pt 1: 43-45.

[10] Formarier M. La qualité de vie pour des personnes ayant un problème de santé. Rech Soins Infirm 2007; 88: 3.

[11] Goodinson SM, Singleton J. Quality of life: a critical review of current concepts, measures and their clinical implications. Int J Nurs Stud 1989; 26: 327-341.

[12] Mallouli M, Dardouri M, Ajmi T, et al. Factors Determining the Quality of Life of Patients With COPD. Clin Pulm Med 2017; 24: 227-231.

[13] Vaske I, Kenn K, Keil DC, et al. Illness perceptions and coping with disease in chronic obstructive pulmonary disease: Effects on health-related quality of life. J Health Psychol 2017; 22: 1570-1581.

[14] Monteagudo M, Rodríguez-Blanco T, Llagostera M, et al. Factors associated with changes in quality of life of COPD patients: A prospective study in primary care. *Respir Med*; 107. Epub ahead of print 2013. DOI: 10.1016/j.rmed.2013.05.009.

[15] Liang L, Lin Y, Yang T, et al. Determinants of health-related quality of life worsening in patients with chronic obstructive pulmonary disease at one year. Chin Med J (Engl) 2014; 127: 4-10.

[16] Lee H, Jhun BW, Cho J, et al. Different impacts of respiratory symptoms and comorbidities on COPD-specific health-related quality of life by COPD severity. *Int J COPD*; 12. Epub ahead of print 2017. DOI: 10.2147/COPD.S145910.

[17] Esteban C, Arostegui I, Aramburu A, et al. Predictive factors

over time of health-related quality of life in COPD patients. *Respir Res*; 21. Epub ahead of print 5 June 2020. DOI: 10.1186/s12931-020-01395-z.

[18] Park SK. Changes in symptoms and health-related quality of life in patients with exacerbated chronic obstructive pulmonary disease. *Appl Nurs Res*; 54. Epub ahead of print 1 August 2020. DOI: 10.1016/j.apnr.2020.151278.

[19] Amini S, Ghasemi A, Solduzian M, et al. Is Inhaler Technique Associated with Quality of Life in Patients with Chronic Obstructive Pulmonary Disease? *Curr Ther Res*; 93. Epub ahead of print 2020. DOI: 10.1016/j.curtheres.2020.100608.

[20] Sundh J, Johansson G, Larsson K, et al. Comorbidity and health-related quality of life in patients with severe chronic obstructive pulmonary disease attending swedish secondary care units. Int J COPD 2015; 10: 173-183.

[21] Kendrová L, Mikuľáková W, Nechvátal P, et al. QUALITY OF LIFE IN PATIENTS WITH CHRONIC OBSTRUCTIVE PULMONARY DISEASE IN SLOVAKIA. Hrvat Rev za Rehabil istraživanja 2015; 51: 57-63.

[22] Deslee G, Burgel PR, Escamilla R, et al. Impact of current cough on health-related quality of life in patients with COPD. Int J COPD 2016; 11: 2091-2097.

[23] Martinez CH, Diaz AA, Parulekar AD, et al. Age-related differences in health-related quality of life in COPD: An analysis of the COPDGene and SPIROMICS Cohorts. Chest 2016; 149: 927-935.

[24] Negi H, Sarkar M, Raval A, et al. Health-related quality of life in patients with chronic obstructive pulmonary disease in North India. J Postgrad Med 2014; 60: 7-11.

[25] Deslee G, Burgel PR, Escamilla R, et al. Impact of current cough on health-related quality of life in patients with COPD. *Int J COPD*; 11. Epub ahead of print 2016. DOI: 10.2147/COPD.S106883.

[26] Brien SB, Stuart B, Dickens AP, et al. Independent determinants of disease-related quality of life in COPD – Scope for nonpharmacologic interventions? *Int J COPD*; 13. Epub ahead of print 2018. DOI: 10.2147/COPD.S152955.

[27] Kwon HY, Kim E. Factors contributing to quality of life in COPD patients in South Korea. *Int J COPD*; 11. Epub ahead of print 2016. DOI: 10.2147/COPD.S90566.

[28] Hammoudeh S, Gadelhaq W, Janahi I. Prospective Cohort Studies in Medical Research. IntechOpen, pp. 11-28.

[29] Mercier M, Schraub S. *Qualité de vie : quels outils de mesure ? Comment mesurer la qualité de vie ?* DaTeBe, Courbevoie (FRA), http://documents.irevues.inist.fr/handle/2042/9760 (2005, accessed 18 February 2021).

[30] Van Manen JG, Bindels PJE, Dekker FW, et al. The influence of COPD on health-related quality of life independent of the influence of comorbidity. J Clin Epidemiol 2003; 56: 1177-1184.

Chapter 5

Exercise Training and Pulmonary Rehabilitation in COPD

Amira Permatasari Tarigan and Fannie Rizki Ananda

Abstract

Systemic inflammation and deconditioning syndrome lead to loss of structural and function of body muscle, particularly in extremity muscle. Longer period of inactivity due to dyspnea worsen the destruction of muscle. Regular and gradually increase exercise training as part of pulmonary rehabilitation (PR) can improve the function of essential muscles in doing daily life so stable Chronic Obstructive Pulmonary Disease (COPD) patient can maintenance their daily activities with minimal limitations. Pulmonary rehabilitation consists of exercise training, nutritional support, smoking cessation, and self-management of COPD. The prescription of exercise training is mandatory. Assessment of clinical condition to adjust the type of training, duration, frequency, and intensity of training must be completed before beginning the training session. Regular and gradually increased training gives significant impact in improving lung function, dyspnea scale, and quality of life in patient with stable COPD. However, in this covid era, the restriction of hospital attending PR was significantly affect PR program. As immunocompromised population, COPD patient have higher risk for COVID19 infection and develops more severe complications compare with normal population. So, the modified supervised and unsupervised training was needed to revise the classic type of PR. Tele-rehabilitation with teleconference, phone calls, and interactive web based PR can be the good alternative in decreasing hospital admission and improving quality of life in patient with COPD.

Keywords: Pulmonary rehabilitation, exercise training, COPD, tele-rehabilitation, covid-era

1. Introduction

Dyspnea is the main symptom of Chronic Obstructive Pulmonary Disease (COPD) that correlates with the limitation of daily activity [1, 2], anxiety and other psychological impacts [3, 4], low quality of life [5], and reduced survival rate [6]. Dyspnea can manifest across the degree of pulmonary obstruction. Either patients with moderate or severe obstruction can experience dyspnea in their daily activities [7]. All these facts cause dyspnea and exercise tolerance becoming the main focus in COPD management in a few guidelines [8, 9].

Besides the pharmacological approach, pulmonary rehabilitation (PR) is considered an important part of comprehensive COPD treatment, particularly in group B-D [10]. Almost all types of pulmonary rehabilitation have a positive impact on the dyspnea scale of patients with COPD. Six-week of pulmonary rehabilitation was given to the end-stage of COPD outpatients and provide a significant improvement of dyspnea scale using a visual analog scale [11]. A meta-analysis study also suggests including upper extremity exercise in pulmonary rehabilitation because it can relieve dyspnea in COPD, although few studies showed the insignificant difference of Borg scale after the training [12]. A study that compares endurance training, combined endurance and strength training, and pharmacological alone showed the improvement of dyspnea in endurance and combined training, but not in a pharmacological alone group. It stated that strength training gives an additional impact on muscle force, but not different from endurance training alone in health status [13]. This is in line with the previous author's study that showed 4 weeks of upper extremity exercise without strength training had demonstrated the improvement of dyspnea scale using the mMRC scale [14].

On the other side, an intervention study with 6 weeks of cardiopulmonary exercise showed an insignificant improvement of dyspnea scale measured with 0–10 Category Ratio (CR) in COPD patients [15]. But as general, a review article that compiles few meta-analyses, randomized controlled study, reviews, and the clinical trial showed that pulmonary rehabilitation gives positive impacts in COPD patients according to functional outcomes, dyspnea scale, and quality of life [16]. Different results might be caused by different dyspnea scales used in the various study. But according to GOLD, the Borg scale and mMRC scale were recommended to measure the dyspnea scale in COPD patients (*Global Initiative for Chronic Obstructive Lung Disease*, 2019).

Breathing training as part of PR can improve regional ventilation and gas exchange and respiratory muscle function that later improves the exercise tolerance and quality of life of patients [17]. Breathing training includes diaphragm breathing, pursed-lip breathing, relaxation technique, and body position [18]. In a study, diaphragm breathing alone and the combination of diaphragm breathing and pursed-lip breathing can reduce the asynchrony of inspiration-expiration ratio and increase lung volume [19]. A study also stated the combination of upper limb training and pursed-lip breathing can decrease dyspnea, improve exercise capacity, and quality of life in patients with stable COPD [14]. Diaphragm breathing (DB) itself improves breathing patterns by coordinating the rib cage muscles and abdominal wall, reduce the activity of the accessory muscle, and lead to improving exercise tolerance [20].

2. Deconditioning syndrome

Decondition syndrome refers to the change in the structure and function of body muscle due to inactivity. This syndrome usually occurred in chronic cardiovascular and lung disease, including Chronic Obstructive Pulmonary Disease (COPD) [21, 22]. This change involved muscle, cardiac, lung, and vascular-related to the history of the disease [23]. This syndrome consisted of three steps:

1. Mild deconditioning: this condition affects normal exercise in which a patient will experience dyspnea and fatigue after doing some exercise include cycling, biking, and swimming.

2. Moderate deconditioning: this condition affects daily activities including walking, shopping, and lifting some goods.

3. Severe conditioning: in this condition, the patient cannot do any activities and just laying on the hospital bed.

Decondition syndrome is a vicious cycle that occurred progressively. The longer the period of inactivity, the more severe the deconditioning will be, and the longer it will take to return to your previous level of functioning [21].

Generally, three basic mechanisms contribute to deconditioning syndrome in chronic pulmonary disease. There is an imbalance between oxygen distributed along with the systemic and respiratory muscles and the amount of oxygen served, muscle dysfunctions include a structural and functional change in extremity and respiratory muscle, and imbalance between ventilation capacity and the amount of ventilation needed for running daily activities [24–26].

The disturbance of exercise capacity may result in systemic manifestation rather than pulmonary disease. Systemic inflammation, hypoxia, and deconditioning syndrome are caused by muscle atrophy and loss of muscle functions [26]. Muscle atrophy occurs when there is an imbalance of protein synthesis due to lower testosterone levels [21, 22] and protein degradation. Increased levels of ubiquitin and TNF-α was seen in several studies [26, 27]. Further, malnutrition, chronic hypoxia, oxidative stress will increase systemic inflammation and muscle disturbance [26].

3. Pulmonary rehabilitation

Pulmonary rehabilitation is a substantial part of comprehensive treatment in COPD in every stage. According to GOLD 2021, pulmonary rehabilitation is recommended in stage B-D of stable COPD. Pulmonary rehabilitation includes exercise training, smoking cessation, nutrition, and education for self-management intervention [28]. Pulmonary rehabilitation should be offered to patients with COPD to improve dyspnoea and health status by a clinically important amount. Besides, pulmonary rehabilitation also alleviates psychological disturbance results in the long-term effect of chronic pulmonary disease.

1. Exercise training

   Exercise training is the main part of pulmonary rehabilitation. According to GOLD 2020, regular exercise training can improve shortness of breath, exercise tolerance, and quality of life status [29]. Exercise training includes endurance/aerobic training, strength training, and inspiratory muscle training. According to GOLD 2021, the combination of these training gives better outcomes compared with the method alone [28].

2. Nutritional support

   In COPD patients, the high level of katabolic cytokines contributed to malnutrition [30]. A high level of IL-6, IL-8, TNF-α showed in COPD patients and their levels have a role as predictors of worse outcomes in COPD [26, 30–32]. Also, high broadcasting of leptin in COPD patient play roles in decreased appetite consequently in decreased muscle mass and functions [33, 34]. Twenty-five to forty percent of COPD patients experienced malnutrition and 25% of them has moderate to severe malnutrition with low fatty fat mass [35].

   The nutritional intervention showed a significant increase in muscle mass and function leads to exercise tolerance improvement. Antioxidant properties in vegetables and fruit may increase the antioxidant resulted in decreasing systemic inflammation [36]. Besides, high fat with low carbohydrate food also showed the improvement of pulmonary function in stable COPD patients [37]. So, after the exercise training intervention, nutritional support must be considered as a substantial part of pulmonary rehabilitation.

3. Self-care management of COPD

   Individual management of COPD is an important part of pulmonary rehabilitation. We have to educate the patient about steps of smoking cessation, an inhaler used, recognition of exacerbation, and when to admit to the hospital. The patient should be known his condition, including the risk and complications of his disease, and the risk of not taking medicine regularly. They should be informed about the factors contributing to exacerbation and how to handle them. In this session, physicians must collaborate not only with the patient but also with his patient's family. Motivate the patient to stop smoking or even changed his job if it contributed to the uncontrolled symptom of COPD. Education also involved how to convincing the patient for taking the exercise training regularly and continue attending the session of exercise training by himself after discharge from the hospital [28].

4. Exercise training preparation

Before beginning the session of training, we must assess the baseline condition of the patient to prepare the individual dose of training.

Following assessment must be undergone for every stable COPD patient [28]:

1. A detailed history and physical examination of the patient. This must be important to rule out the group of the patient and the risk for exacerbation.

2. Measurement of airway obstruction using spirometer before and after bronchodilator

3. Assessment of exercise capacity using the six-minute walking test. In the available facilities, cycle ergometer and treadmill exercise can be used to measure the physiological variables that impact the exercise capacity, including maximum oxygen consumption, maximum heart rate, and maximum work performed [28].

4. Health status and the impact of breathlessness in doing exercise

5. Assessing the respiratory and limb muscle in patients with muscle wasting

6. Individual patient goals and expectations

4.1 Prescription of exercise training in COPD

There are few parameters must be considered to prescribe an exercise training in COPD patient. There was no guideline plainly stated that exercise training cannot be done in an exacerbated state. The frequency, intensity, time, and type of exercise training, abbreviate by FITT must be reviewed before beginning the session of training. And these parameters also correlated with outcomes [29].

According to one systematic review, there was dose-related training and outcomes. High-intensity training tends to have more significance to exercise tolerance measured by maximal heart rate and oxygen uptake in exercise (VO2max) [38]. But the problem is the practical and economic reasons, the duration of lasting longer than 6–8 weeks of supervised training considered to highly economic demands [39] considered to be significant. According to consensus, exercise training is arranged for 6–12 weeks duration with two to three supervised sessions per week with 60–90 minutes for 1 session [39–42].

4.2 Frequency of supervised training

1. Exercise training programs should be two-five times a week [39, 43]

2. Supervised of pulmonary rehabilitation should be minimum 2 times a week, other sessions can be undergone at home without supervised by physicians or therapist

4.3 Duration of supervised training

1. 30 minutes of physical activity gives a positive impact on a healthy subject [39, 43]

2. 6–12 weeks of training are recommended in all types of exercise training.

3. Long term training (more than six months of training) for outpatient give a more significant impact on exercise tolerance, exacerbation events, and quality of life [44]

4. Intermittent exercise can be arranged for a patient who cannot tolerate continuous training. In initial training, moderate to severe COPD tend to have only a few minutes of training and we can increase it gradually by about 5–10 minutes every 1–2 weeks [45].

4.4 Intensity of training

1. 50–80% maximal workload must be arranged in exercise. According to American Sports Medicine, it is divided into [45]:

   Light intensity: 30–40% peak work rate.

   Vigorous-intensity: 60–80% peak work rate

2. American Thoracic Society and European Respiratory Society recommend initial training with >60% maximal work rate [40].

3. Workload defined as VO2 max and maximum heart rate with the formula is 220-age

4. Targeted of intensity is 60–70% RM (Repetition Maximum) or 100% of 8–12 RM

5. American Association of Cardiovascular and Pulmonary Rehabilitation (AACRP) recommended initiating the training with light intensity and gradually increased it until reaches the maximal target [46].

4.5 Type of training

1. Endurance training

   Endurance training is the most common training prescribed for severe COPD. Endurance training can improve aerobic exercise capacity so the patient can do his daily activities more comfortably without shortness of breath [47]. Endurance training also can improve peripheral muscle function in severe COPD patients [48]. But according to the Casaburi study, endurance training with high intensity has a greater impact compared with low intensity [22]. But this intensity can be gradually increased in line with the patient's condition. Walking and cycling are the most recommended endurance training for exercising the lower limb [49]. Fatigue in large muscles in the thigh including quadriceps femur muscle and hamstring muscle often occurs at the beginning of the training [50, 51]. But, it will decrease after a few sessions of training, so a gradually increased dose is needed in the training arrangement. Further, walking on the ground give a more significant impact in improving the walking capacity in severe COPD patients [49]. Upper extremity exercise involved biceps, triceps, deltoid, and accessory respiratory muscles including latissimus dorsi muscle and pectoralis mayor should be trained to give additional effect in alleviating shortness of breath [14].

A six-minutes walking test (6-MWT) is the most recommended examination for assessing the impact of endurance training [39]. Due to its economic aspect, easy to do, low side effect, 6-mwt is recommended in every guideline [39, 40]. But, a cardiopulmonary exercise test (CPET) has been a gold standard in assessing exercise capacity. We can measure cardiorespiratory performance and VO2 max [45]. However, this method is expensive and needs more equipment so it cannot be done performed in every facility, particularly in healthcare facilities without a standard pulmonary rehabilitation center. Other measures can sit to stand tests (STST), incremental shuttle walking test (ISWT), and endurance shuttle walking test (ESWT) [49].

2. Strength training

Disturbance of muscle structure and function in COPD patients has been discussed before. Strength training or resistance training give a more significant impact on muscle enhancement in COPD patients [40, 42, 47]. Its impact in peripheral and large muscle alleviate dyspnea and improving the activity which gives more effort including climbing the stairs, standing, and arm elevation [47]. So, if combining with endurance training, a systematic review shows a greater impact on the quality of life of a patient with COPD [52].

Frequency, intensity, repetition, and type of strength training contribute to the impact of training. Large individual variations further affect the quality of training. Six until twelve repetitions about 15–45 minutes for 2–3 days recommended in strength training in some guidelines [41]. The patient can take a break when begin to experience dyspnea. A short bronchodilator should be given immediately with oxygen supplementation.

3. Inspiratory muscle training

Different from endurance and strength training, inspiratory muscle training focused on the enhancement of the diaphragm [17]. In COPD, the emphysema process made the disturbance of the elasticity of the diaphragm to make contraction and relaxation, showed in the hyperinflated lung, narrowed and more vertical heart, and flattened diaphragm in radiographic appearance.

Inspiratory muscle training improves diaphragm muscle strength and endurance so it can reduce dyspnea [47]. This training is often combined with upper and lower body training for maximizing the effect of pulmonary rehabilitation in stable COPD.

This training was recommended in 5–7 days per week with a duration 7x2 minutes interval approach and 1-minute rest between intervals. The total duration of this training is 15–20 minutes for each day [53, 54].

4.6 Variation of exercise training

There is no absolute content of exercise training in COPD. We can design our method according to our facilities and human resources. In our setting, we have arranged a few methods of exercise training and showed a significant impact on breathing scale and quality of life.

Below is one of the type of exercise training in our setting. The procedures include:

After taken the baseline data, patients in the intervention group were scheduled for the training program. The training program was held twice a week for four weeks. The procedures of the study were the following:

1. Heating. Participants were given infrared radiation for 10 minutes in their chest to warm the chest muscle and facilitate sputum expectorant.

2. Chest therapy. In this session, the chest muscle was massaged, stretched, and then vibrated to facilitate the sputum expectorant.

3. Upper limb endurance training with simple gymnastics using the neck, shoulder, and arm. Along with these procedures, pursed-lip breathing was performed to facilitate breathing training

4. Upper limb strength training using dumbbell with personalized weight lifting. First, we examined the maximal weight lifting in five repetitions. For the 1st week of practice, we used 60% of maximal weight lifting (kg) and then increased progressively every week.

Upper limb endurance training in our setting consisted of few 10 moves (**Figures 1–10**):

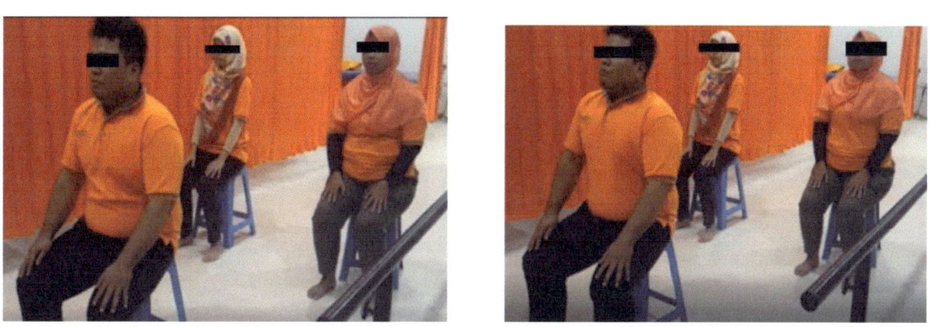

Figure 1.
Pursed lip breathing with exhaling while tilting your head towards your shoulder.

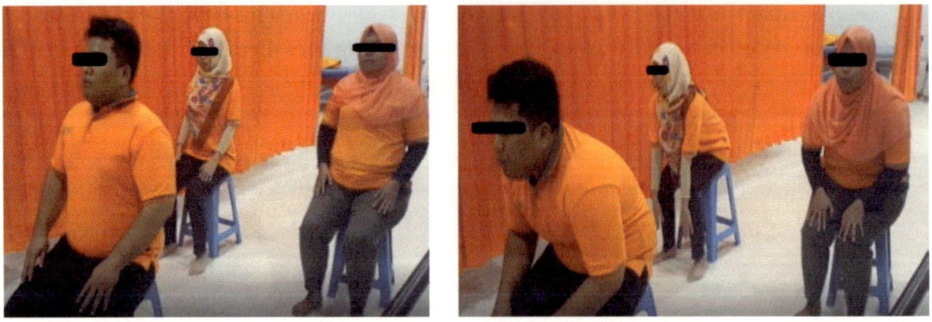

Figure 2.
Bird-like pattern with inhaling while body straightening, exhale while bending forward to the bottom.

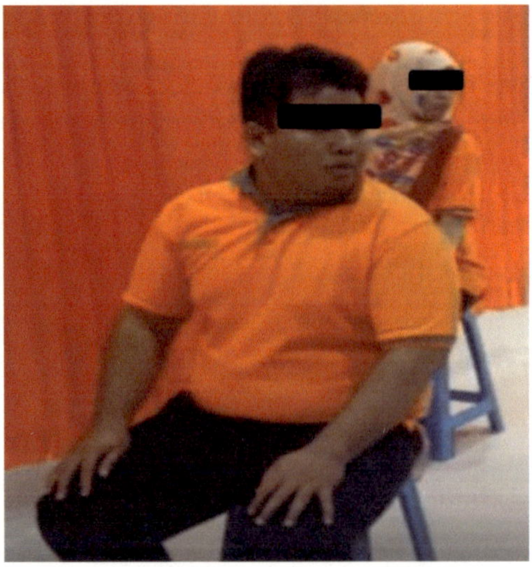

Figure 3.
No-way pattern with pursed-lip breathing, seeing movement to left and right alternately.

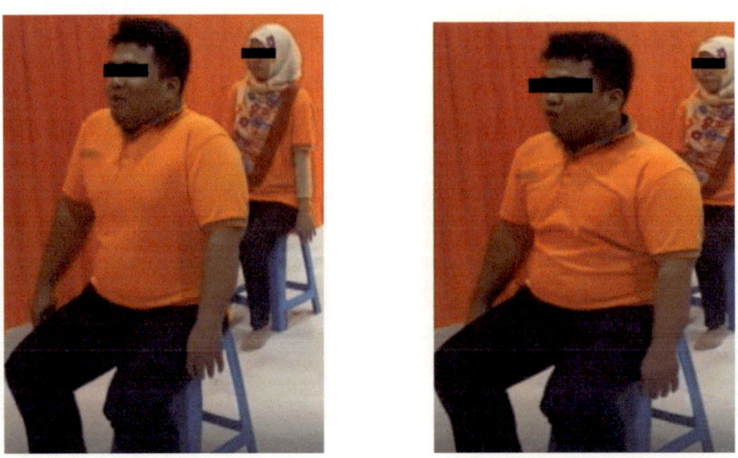

Figure 4.
Shoulder shrug with pursed-lip breathing.

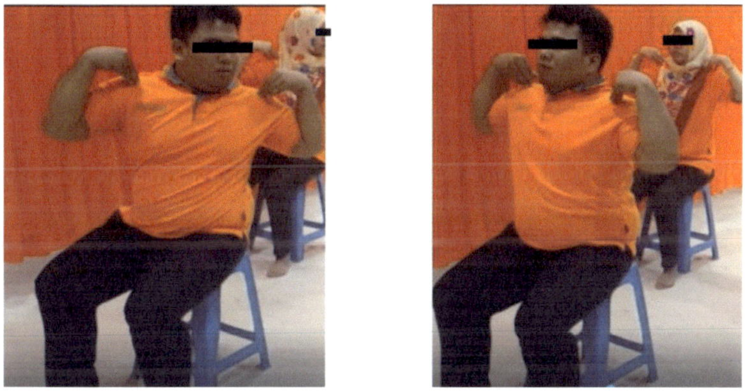

Figure 5.
Fan-like movement with pursed-lip breathing, hands are bent together, then turn right and left.

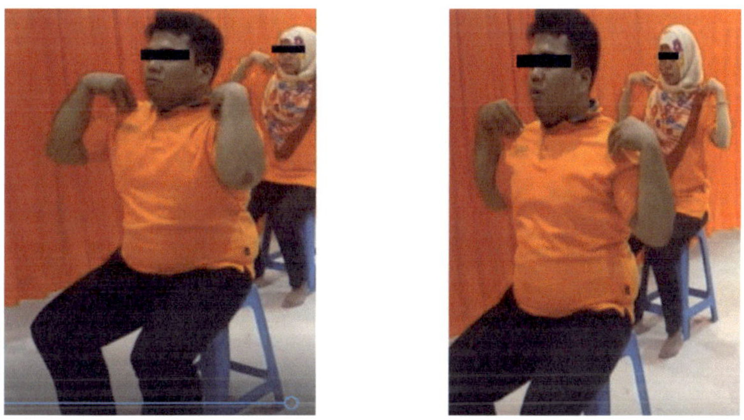

Figure 6.
Chicken cuckoo like movements with rotating the shoulder with hands bent at the shoulder.

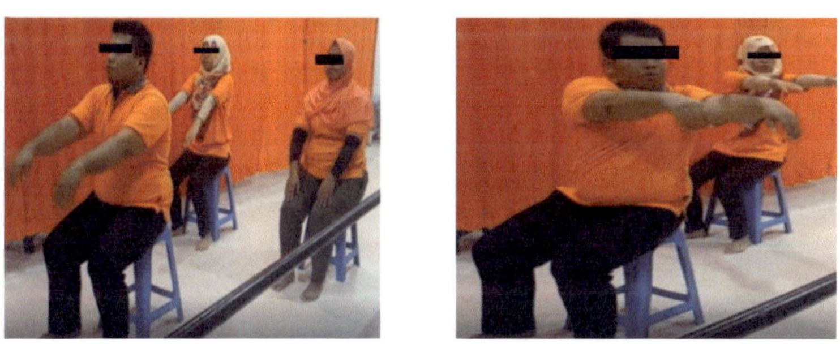

Figure 7.
Vampire-like movement, hands straight forward while inhaling, then rotating the body to the right, left, and forwards while exhaling.

5. Supported vs. unsupported pulmonary rehabilitation

Long-term PR tends to gradually decrease over a while [55]. Many circumstances contribute to discontinuous training after a short period of intensive PR, including lack of motivation, support from friends and families, disease progressivity, and distance from health facilities [56]. For the last reason, home-based PR might become

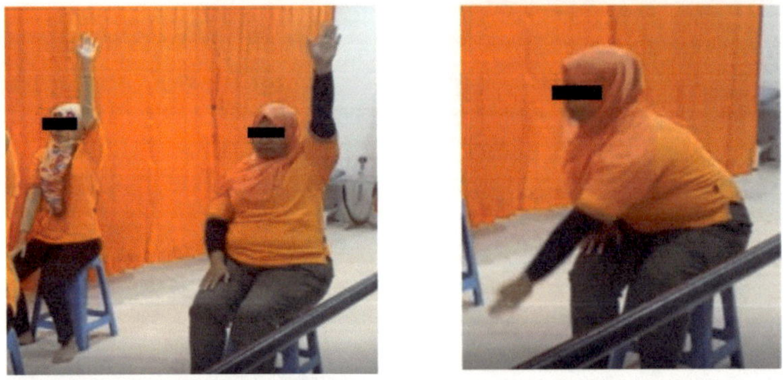

Figure 8.
Calling movement, the hand is lifted, then touched downwards, in the opposite direction.

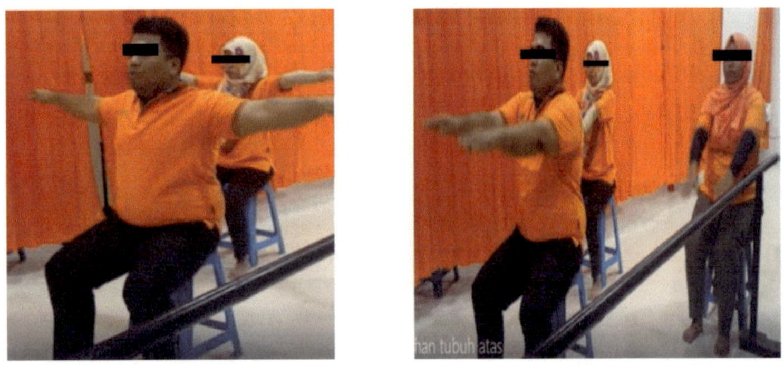

Figure 9.
Butterfly-like pattern, hands stretched straight forward then hands stretch.

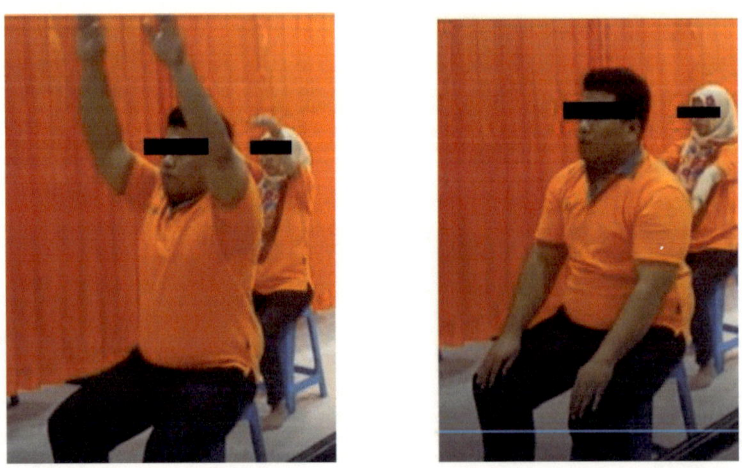

Figure 10.
Cooling down with pursed lip breathing.

an alternative. According to Swerts et al., the continuation of 12 weeks of supervised training maintained 1-year of walking ability in stable COPD patients [57]. Further, Ries et al. suggested a year of home-based PR with once a month of supervised training at health facilities to control the procedure and the impact of PR in the stable COPD patient. Ries et al. also evaluate the impact of maintenance PR by telephone for

1 year after a short period of supervised training in health care facilities. This study revealed that during the first 12 months, there were improvements in exercise tolerance and health status in patients undergone telephone supervised training and once in a month controlled training at health facilities in chronic pulmonary disease [58].

There were no definite guidelines that recommend the duration of supported and unsupported PR. But studies showed that 8–12 weeks of supported PR followed by 12–24 months of giving substantial effect in exercise tolerance and quality of life in a patient with COPD [56]. In another study, Guel et al. showed that 6 months of intensive supervised training followed by 6 months of once-in-week supervised exercise training give an improvement of dyspnea scale and quality of life compared with the control group which no additional PR after intensive supervised training [59]. Another study also showed the reduction of exacerbation with hospital admission after retreatment PR in outpatient with stable chronic pulmonary disease who has stopped PR for 1 year, although there was no difference in exercise tolerance and quality of life compare with the control group [60].

There are few modifications for unsupported PR. We can monitor once a week or once a month to control the correct procedure and the impact that might be occurred, both positive and negative impact.

More than 50% of the participant who attends long term PR was a loss to follow up. Both once in a month or once in three months of supervised training with the rest session is home-based PR showed no significant difference in the 1-year loss to follow up [61]. Whereas, the impact of intensive and supervised PR for 8–12 weeks will disappear after 1 year [56]. So, the long-term supported PR is needed to improve the exercise capacity and dyspnea tolerance in stable COPD patients to maintain their daily life.

6. Tele-rehabilitation in Covid19 era

In this pandemic era, pulmonary rehabilitation was significantly affected. Strict regulation to decrease hospital admission in people with COPD gives a significant impact on stable COPD patients who attend regular pulmonary rehabilitation in the hospital [62]. Further, COPD patients were susceptible to infections due to lack of immunity and chronic inflammatory state. So, a new era of pulmonary rehabilitation was needed to reform the classic pulmonary rehabilitation.

Theoretically, teleconference PR will enhance the adherence to attending PR sessions in stable COPD patients, particularly patients whose address was far from the PR center. But, data showed that there was no significant difference in the impact of a patient who attends teleconference PR compare with conventional PR [62]. Few factors contribute to the poor adherence to PR programs. They are including availability, accessibility, and attrition [63]. The alternative method including home-based supervision, interactive web-based PR, videoconference with telehealth can be implicated in the new settings of PR [64–66].

Teleconference PR or telerehabilitation has been discussed since early 2000. Tele-rehabilitation was the new concept of PR where the patient was being at home and used communication and information to provide PR [67]. This was promising alternative ways in patients whose addresses were far from the PR center and in this covid era. On the other side, this alternative way also has severe limitations including short duration of intervention, small patient number, communication error, limitation of technology facilities, and poor adherence of several components of PR [65]. Specific guidelines of telerehabilitation must be accomplished to achieve maximal impact on the patient. This needs the coordination of several aspects including administration, organization, physical trainee, physicians, and government [67].

In telerehabilitation particularly in chronic respiratory disease, few modules must be carried out. Inhaler used training, smoking cessation, dietary and self-management advice, physical exercise, and psychological support must be scheduled formally through phone calls or video conference with a certain physiotherapist, dietician, and pulmonologist [66, 68]. There were no guidelines regulate the definite duration, frequency, and type of training in telerehabilitation. Bhatt study arranges 36 exercise sessions in 12 weeks consists of a combination of stretching and breathing training for warming up, aerobic exercise including ergometer bicycles until maximum heart rate was achieved (60–80% maximal HR). Resistance training used resistance band was performed with a video tutorial that was given before. Also, breathing training including basic yoga training, diaphragm breathing training, paced-training, and pursed-lip breathing was carried out in stable COPD patients. After few sessions, an educational video conference was performed consisted of smoking cessation, psychological support, appropriate inhaler technique, disease education, monitoring, and reporting exacerbation [66]. Another study performed 144 sessions for 12 months with 2 months of initial training PR programs in the PR center to educate the patients to use the modal facilities and how to monitor the function of each piece of equipment. In the next 10 months, patients were undergone self-exercise training with remote monitoring. Educational programs including dietary, self-management, and psychological support were performed in a video conference. Strict monitoring of vital signs during training particularly heart rate and oxygen saturation were recorded and send to physicians after the end of each training session [68]. After all the training session, several parameters can be measured to evaluate the impact of the teleconference, including modified Medical Research Council dyspnoea scale (mMRC), COPD assessment questionnaire (CAT), St. George's Respiratory Questionnaire (SGRQ), Hospital Anxiety and Depression Scale (HADS), spirometer, pedometer, and hospitalization event, length of stay, and Emergency Room visits [66, 68].

Few studies have proved that telerehabilitation has benefits to stable COPD patients. Bhatt's study showed that early telerehabilitation after the patient was discharged from the hospital due to exacerbation has reduced 30 days of re-admission in hospital from all causes of exacerbation [66]. Vasiloupoulou's study also stated that home-based maintenance telerehabilitation was the same effect as hospital-based PR in reducing the risk of acute exacerbation and hospitalization [68].

New South Wales Health of Ministry has arranged telehealth pulmonology rehabilitation in the covid19 era. It consisted of four main components including patient assessment by phone calls and teleconference, home-based individual exercise program by videoconferencing, patient education, and the re-assessment of the patient after completed all the training programs [69].

1. Patient assessment

   Phone calls and video conferences can be conducted in the patient assessment sessions. It is included general medical history contains respiratory symptoms, social history, the course of the disease, history of hospitalization, medication, vaccinations, and smoking history. Symptoms were evaluated by Borg scale, mMRC, SGRQ, CAT, HADS, and CRQ. Objective measurement must be carried out including height, weight, oxygen saturation, blood pressure, and heart rate. Further, lower limb strength can be measured by 5 minutes sit to stand test (5STS) while lower limb endurance is measured by a 1-minute sit to stand test (1STS).

2. Exercise programs

   There are few types of telehealth PR. NSW Health recommends lower limb endurance training using the walking method while the endurance training by

5STS and squats-stand. Upper limb training used light hand weights for endurance training and a resistance band for strength training.

a. Duration: lower limb endurance (start 10–15 minutes and continue in 30 minutes); upper limb endurance (10 mins); lower limb strength (10 mins); upper limb strength (10 mins)

b. Intensity: moderate to severe

c. Frequency: 2 days in PR center and other 2 days at home

d. Length of programs: 8 weeks

e. Type: continues, interval, and intermittent

3. Patient education

   a. Description about lung disease

   b. The benefit of exercise programs and physical activity

   c. Symptom evaluation and management

   d. Inhaler technique

   e. Smoking cessation

   f. Nutrition

   g. Psychological support

4. Re-assessment

7. Conclusions

Last, COPD patient was advised to follow the pulmonary rehabilitation to do exercise training by themselves. Pulmonary rehabilitation is comprehensive management and evaluation that involved a few basic knowledge including nutrition, psychologist, physiotherapist, pulmonologist, and other specialist doctors depend on the patient's condition and co-morbid.

Author details

Amira Permatasari Tarigan[1*] and Fannie Rizki Ananda[2]

1 Asthma and COPD Division, Department of Pulmonology and Respiratory Medicine, Faculty of Medicine, Universitas Sumatera Utara, Indonesia

2 Department of Pulmonology and Respiratory Medicine, Faculty of Medicine, Universitas Sumatera Utara, Indonesia

*Address all correspondence to: amira@usu.ac.id

References

[1] O'Donnell DE, Laveneziana P. Dyspnea and activity limitation in COPD: mechanical factors. COPD [Internet]. 2007 Sep [cited 2019 Aug 21];4(3):225-36. Available from: http://www.ncbi.nlm.nih.gov/pubmed/17729066

[2] Roche N. Activity limitation: A major consequence of dyspnoea in COPD. European Respiratory Review. 2009 Jun 1;18(112):54-57.

[3] Yohannes AM, Junkes-Cunha M, Smith J, Vestbo J. Management of Dyspnea and Anxiety in Chronic Obstructive Pulmonary Disease: A Critical Review. Vol. 18, Journal of the American Medical Directors Association. Elsevier Inc.; 2017. p. 1096.e1-1096.e17.

[4] Gianjoppe-Santos J, Sentanin AC, Barusso MS, Rizzatti FPG, Jamami M, Pires Di Lorenzo VA. Impact of exacerbation of COPD on anxiety and depression symptoms and dyspnea in the activities of daily living. In European Respiratory Society (ERS); 2015. p. PA3306.

[5] Anzueto A, Miravitlles M. Pathophysiology of dyspnea in COPD. Postgrad Med [Internet]. 2017 Apr [cited 2019 Aug 21];129(3):366-74. Available from: http://www.ncbi.nlm.nih.gov/pubmed/28277858

[6] Lange P, Marott JL, Vestbo J, Nordestgaard BG. Prevalence of night-time dyspnoea in COPD and its implications for prognosis. Eur Respir J. 2014;43(6):1590-1598.

[7] O'Donnell DE, Elbehairy AF, Faisal A, Webb KA, Neder JA, Mahler DA. Exertional dyspnoea in COPD: The clinical utility of cardiopulmonary exercise testing. Eur Respir Rev. 2016 Sep 1;25(141):333-347.

[8] O'Donnell DE, Hernandez P, Kaplan A, Aaron S, Bourbeau J, Marciniuk D, et al. CTS COPD Highlights. Can Respir J [Internet]. 2008 [cited 2019 Aug 21];15 Suppl A(February):1A-8A. Available from: http://www.pubmedcentral.nih.gov/articlerender.fcgi?artid=2802325&tool=pmcentrez&rendertype=abstract

[9] Qaseem A, Wilt TJ, Weinberger SE, Hanania NA, Criner G, van der Molen T, et al. Diagnosis and management of stable chronic obstructive pulmonary disease: a clinical practice guideline update from the American College of Physicians, American College of Chest Physicians, American Thoracic Society, and European Respiratory Society. Ann Intern Med [Internet]. 2011 Aug 2 [cited 2019 Aug 21];155(3):179-91. Available from: http://www.ncbi.nlm.nih.gov/pubmed/21810710

[10] Global Initiative for Chronic Obstructive L ung D isease [Internet]. 2019 [cited 2019 Jun 10]. Available from: www.goldcopd.org

[11] Ngaage DL, Hasney K, Cowen ME. The functional impact of an individualized, graded, outpatient pulmonary rehabilitation in end-stage chronic obstructive pulmonary disease. 1 Ngaage DL, Hasney K, Cowen ME Funct impact an Individ graded, outpatient Pulm Rehabil end-stage chronic Obstr Pulm Dis Hear Lung [Internet] [cited 2019 Mar 4];33(6)381-9 Available from http// www [Internet]. [cited 2019 Mar 4];33(6):381-9. Available from: http://www.ncbi.nlm.nih.gov/pubmed/15597292

[12] Pan L, Guo YZ, Yan JH, Zhang WX, Sun J, Li BW. Does upper extremity exercise improve dyspnea in patients with COPD? A meta-analysis. Respir Med [Internet]. 2012 Nov [cited 2019 Mar 4];106(11):1517-25. Available from:

http://www.ncbi.nlm.nih.gov/pubmed/22902265

[13] Daabis R, Hassan M, Zidan M. Endurance and strength training in pulmonary rehabilitation for COPD patients. Egypt J Chest Dis Tuberc. 2017 Apr;66(2):231-236.

[14] Tarigan AP, Ananda FR, Pandia P, Sinaga BYM, Maryaningsih M, Anggriani A. The Impact of Upper Limb Training with Breathing Maneuver in Lung Function , Functional Capacity , Dyspnea Scale , and Quality of Life in Patient with Stable Chronic Obstructive of Lung Disease. Open access Maced J Med Sci [Internet]. 2019 Feb 28 [cited 2019 Mar 26];7(4):567-72. Available from: http://www.ncbi.nlm.nih.gov/pubmed/30894913

[15] Mahler DA, Ward J, Mejia-Alfaro R. Stability of dyspnea ratings after exercise training in patients with COPD. Med Sci Sports Exerc. 2003 Jul 1;35(7):1083-1087.

[16] Santus P, Bassi L, Radovanovic D, Airoldi A, Raccanelli R, Triscari F, et al. Pulmonary Rehabilitation in COPD: A Reappraisal (2008-2012). Pulm Med [Internet]. 2013 [cited 2019 Mar 5];2013:374283. Available from: http://www.ncbi.nlm.nih.gov/pubmed/23365741

[17] Gosselink R. REVIEW SERIES: physiotherapy techniques for respiratory disease Breathing techniques in patients with chronic obstructive pulmonary disease (COPD) [Internet]. Vol. 1, Chronic Respiratory Disease. 2004. Available from: www.CRDjournal.com

[18] Borge CR, Hagen KB, Mengshoel AM, Omenaas E, Moum T, Wahl AK. Effects of controlled breathing exercises and respiratory muscle training in people with chronic obstructive pulmonary disease: Results from evaluating the quality of evidence in systematic reviews. BMC Pulm Med. 2014 Nov 21;14(1).

[19] Mendes LPS, Moraes KS, Hoffman M, Vieira DSR, Ribeiro-Samora GA, Lage SM, et al. Effects of diaphragmatic breathing with and without pursed-lips breathing in subjects with COPD. Respir Care. 2019 Feb 1;64(2):136-144.

[20] Fernandes M, Cukier A, Feltrim MIZ. Efficacy of diaphragmatic breathing in patients with chronic obstructive pulmonary disease. Chron Respir Dis. 2011 Nov;8(4):237-244.

[21] Casaburi R. Impacting patient-centred outcomes in COPD: Deconditioning. In: European Respiratory Review. 2006. p. 42-6.

[22] Casaburi R, Porszasz J, Burns MR, Carithers ER, Chang RS, Cooper CB. Physiologic benefits of exercise training in rehabilitation of patients with severe chronic obstructive pulmonary disease. Am J Respir Crit Care Med [Internet]. 1997 May [cited 2019 May 31];155(5):1541-51. Available from: http://www.ncbi.nlm.nih.gov/pubmed/9154855

[23] Crisafulli E, Costi S, Fabbri LM, Clini EM. Respiratory muscles training in COPD patients. Vol. 2, International Journal of COPD. 2007. p. 19-25.

[24] Gea J, Casadevall C, Pascual S, Orozco-Levi M, Barreiro E. Respiratory diseases and muscle dysfunction. Vol. 6, Expert Review of Respiratory Medicine. 2012. p. 75-90.

[25] Pleguezuelos E, Esquinas C, Moreno E, Guirao L, Ortiz J, Garcia-Alsina J, et al. Muscular Dysfunction in COPD: Systemic Effect or Deconditioning? Lung [Internet]. 2016 Apr 1 [cited 2020 Dec 20];194(2):249-57. Available from: https://link.springer.com/article/10.1007/s00408-015-9838-z

[26] Ci R, Degens WH. Factors contributing to muscle wasting and

dysfunction in COPD patients. Vol. 2007, International Journal of COPD. 2007.

[27] Reid MB, Li YP. Tumor necrosis factor α and muscle wasting: A cellular perspective. Respir Res [Internet]. 2001 Jul 12 [cited 2020 Dec 20];2(5):269-72. Available from: https://link.springer.com/articles/10.1186/rr67

[28] 2021 GOLD Reports - Global Initiative for Chronic Obstructive Lung Disease - GOLD [Internet]. [cited 2020 Dec 11]. Available from: https://goldcopd.org/2021-gold-reports/

[29] Patel S, Maddocks M, London WD, Man -C, Harefield P, Respiratory H. Exercise Training in COPD FITT for Purpose? 2020 [cited 2020 Dec 26]; Available from: https://doi.org/10.1016/j.chest.2020.02.040

[30] Rawal G, Yadav S. Nutrition in chronic obstructive pulmonary disease: A review. J Transl Intern Med [Internet]. 2016 Dec 5 [cited 2020 Dec 20];3(4):151-4. Available from: /pmc/articles/PMC4936454/?report=abstract

[31] Gan WQ, Man SFP, Senthilselvan A, Sin DD. Association between chronic obstructive pulmonary disease and systemic inflammation: A systematic review and a meta-analysis [Internet]. Vol. 59, Thorax. Thorax; 2004 [cited 2020 Dec 20]. p. 574-80. Available from: https://pubmed.ncbi.nlm.nih.gov/15223864/

[32] De Godoy I, Donahoe M, Calhoun WJ, Mancino J, Rogers RM. Elevated TNF-α production by peripheral blood monocytes of weight-losing COPD patients. Am J Respir Crit Care Med [Internet]. 1996 [cited 2020 Dec 20];153(2):633-7. Available from: https://pubmed.ncbi.nlm.nih.gov/8564110/

[33] Engelen MPKJ, Schols AMWJ, Baken WC, Wesseling GJ, Wouters EFM. Nutritional depletion in relation to respiratory and peripheral skeletal muscle function in out-patients with COPD. Eur Respir J [Internet]. 1994 [cited 2020 Dec 20];7(10):1793-7. Available from: https://pubmed.ncbi.nlm.nih.gov/7828687/

[34] Mador MJ, Bozkanat E. Skeletal muscle dysfunction in chronic obstructive pulmonary disease. Respir Res [Internet]. 2001 May 2 [cited 2020 Dec 20];2(4):216-24. Available from: http://respiratory-research.biomedcentral.com/articles/10.1186/rr60

[35] Vermeeren MAP, Creutzberg EC, Schols AMWJ, Postma DS, Pieters WR, Roldaan AC, et al. Prevalence of nutritional depletion in a large out-patient population of patients with COPD. Respir Med [Internet]. 2006 Aug [cited 2020 Dec 20];100(8):1349-55. Available from: https://pubmed.ncbi.nlm.nih.gov/16412624/

[36] Shaheen SO, Jameson KA, Syddall HE, Aihie Sayer A, Dennison EM, Cooper C, et al. The relationship of dietary patterns with adult lung function and COPD. Eur Respir J [Internet]. 2010 Aug 1 [cited 2020 Dec 20];36(2):277-84. Available from: www.erj.ersjournals.com

[37] Cai B, Zhu Y, Ma Y, Xu Z, Zao Y, Wang J, et al. Effect of supplementing a high-fat, low-carbohydrate enteral formula in COPD patients. Nutrition. 2003 Mar 1;19(3):229-232.

[38] HSIEH M-J, LAN C-C, CHEN N-H, HUANG C-C, WU Y-K, CHO H-Y, et al. Effects of high-intensity exercise training in a pulmonary rehabilitation programme for patients with chronic obstructive pulmonary disease. Respirology [Internet]. 2007 May [cited 2019 Mar 4];12(3):381-8. Available from: http://www.ncbi.nlm.nih.gov/pubmed/17539842

[39] Bolton CE, Bevan-Smith EF, Blakey JD, Crowe P, Elkin SL, Garrod R, et al. British Thoracic Society guideline on pulmonary rehabilitation in adults [Internet]. Vol. 68, Thorax. BMJ Publishing Group Ltd; 2013 [cited 2020 Dec 26]. p. ii1-30. Available from: http://thorax.bmj.com/

[40] Spruit MA, Singh SJ, Garvey C, Zu Wallack R, Nici L, Rochester C, et al. An official American thoracic society/ European respiratory society statement: Key concepts and advances in pulmonary rehabilitation. Am J Respir Crit Care Med [Internet]. 2013 Oct 15 [cited 2019 Nov 9];188(8). Available from: https://pubmed.ncbi.nlm.nih.gov/24127811/

[41] Nici L, Donner C, Wouters E, Zuwallack R, Ambrosino N, Bourbeau J, et al. American thoracic society/ European respiratory society statement on pulmonary rehabilitation [Internet]. Vol. 173, American Journal of Respiratory and Critical Care Medicine. Am J Respir Crit Care Med; 2006 [cited 2020 Dec 26]. p. 1390-413. Available from: https://pubmed.ncbi.nlm.nih.gov/16760357/

[42] Ries AL, Bauldoff GS, Carlin BW, Casaburi R, Emery CF, Mahler DA, et al. Pulmonary rehabilitation: Joint ACCP/ AACVPR Evidence-Based Clinical Practice Guidelines. Chest [Internet]. 2007 [cited 2020 Dec 26];131(5 SUPPL.):4S-42S. Available from: https://pubmed.ncbi.nlm.nih.gov/17494825/

[43] Morris NR, Walsh J, Adams L, Alision J. Exercise training in COPD: What is it about intensity? Respirology [Internet]. 2016 Oct 1 [cited 2020 Dec 26];21(7):1185-92. Available from: http://doi.wiley.com/10.1111/resp.12864

[44] Zwick RH, Burghuber OC, Dovjak N, Hartl S, Kössler W, Lichtenschopf A, et al. Der Effekt von einem Jahr ambulanter pneumologischer Rehabilitation auf Patienten mit COPD. Wien Klin Wochenschr [Internet]. 2009 Mar [cited 2020 Dec 26];121(5-6):189-95. Available from: https://pubmed.ncbi.nlm.nih.gov/19412748/

[45] ACSMs Guidelines for Exercise Testing and Prescription [Internet]. [cited 2020 Dec 26]. Available from: https://www.acsm.org/read-research/books/acsms-guidelines-for-exercise-testing-and-prescription

[46] Garvey C, Bayles MP, Hamm LF, Hill K, Holland A, Limberg TM, et al. Pulmonary Rehabilitation Exercise Prescription in Chronic Obstructive Pulmonary Disease: Review of Selected Guidelines: An official statement from the American association of cardiovascular and pulmonary rehabilitation. J Cardiopulm Rehabil Prev. 2016;36(2):75-83.

[47] Gloeckl R, Marinov B, Pitta F. Practical recommendations for exercise training in patients with COPD. Eur Respir Rev [Internet]. 2013 Jun 1 [cited 2019 Jun 11];22(128):178-86. Available from: http://err.ersjournals.com/cgi/doi/10.1183/09059180.00000513

[48] Vogiatzis I, Terzis G, Nanas S, Stratakos G, Simoes DCM, Georgiadou O, et al. Skeletal muscle adaptations to interval training in patients with advanced COPD. Chest [Internet]. 2005 Dec 1 [cited 2020 Dec 28];128(6):3838-45. Available from: http://journal.chestnet.org/article/S0012369215496254/fulltext

[49] Zeng Y, Jiang F, Chen Y, Chen P, Cai S. Exercise assessments and trainings of pulmonary rehabilitation in COPD: a literature review. Int J Chron Obstruct Pulmon Dis [Internet]. 2018 Jun 26 [cited 2020 Dec 28];Volume 13:2013-23. Available from: https://www.dovepress.com/exercise-assessments-and-trainings-of-pulmonary-rehabilitation-in-copd-peer-reviewed-article-COPD

[50] Gimeno-Santos E, Rodriguez DA, Barberan-Garcia A, Blanco I, Vilaró J, Torralba Y, et al. Endurance exercise training improves heart rate recovery in patients with COPD. COPD J Chronic Obstr Pulm Dis [Internet]. 2014 [cited 2020 Dec 28];11(2):190-6. Available from: https://pubmed.ncbi.nlm.nih.gov/24377907/

[51] Iepsen UW, Munch GDW, Rugbjerg M, Rinnov AR, Zacho M, Mortensen SP, et al. Effect of endurance versus resistance training on quadriceps muscle dysfunction in COPD: A pilot study. Int J COPD [Internet]. 2016 Oct 27 [cited 2020 Dec 28];11(1):2659-69. Available from: https://pubmed.ncbi.nlm.nih.gov/27822028/

[52] POCKET GUIDE TO COPD DIAGNOSIS, MANAGEMENT, AND PREVENTION A Guide for Health Care Professionals [Internet]. 2020 [cited 2020 Jan 21]. Available from: www.goldcopd.org

[53] Gosselink R, De Vos J, Van Den Heuvel SP, Segers J, Decramer M, Kwakkel G. Impact of inspiratory muscle training in patients with COPD: What is the evidence? [Internet]. Vol. 37, European Respiratory Journal. Eur Respir J; 2011 [cited 2020 Dec 28]. p. 416-25. Available from: https://pubmed.ncbi.nlm.nih.gov/21282809/

[54] Hill K, Jenkins SC, Philippe DL, Cecins N, Shepherd KL, Green DJ, et al. High-intensity inspiratory muscle training in COPD. Eur Respir J [Internet]. 2006 Jun [cited 2020 Dec 28];27(6):1119-28. Available from: https://pubmed.ncbi.nlm.nih.gov/16772388/

[55] Rochester CL. Exercise training in chronic obstructive pulmonary disease [Internet]. Vol. 40, Journal of Rehabilitation Research and Development. [cited 2019 Feb 25]. Available from: https://www.rehab.research.va.gov/jour/03/40/5Sup2/pdf/Rochester.pdf

[56] Gosselink R. Respiratory rehabilitation: Improvement of short- and long-term outcome [Internet]. Vol. 20, European Respiratory Journal. European Respiratory Society; 2002 [cited 2021 Mar 14]. p. 4-5. Available from: https://erj.ersjournals.com/content/20/1/4

[57] Swerts PMJ, Kretzers LMJ, Terpstra-Lindeman E, Verstappen FTJ, Wouters EFM. Exercise reconditioning in the rehabilitation of patients with chronic obstructive pulmonary disease: A short- and long-term analysis. Arch Phys Med Rehabil [Internet]. 1990 Jul 1 [cited 2021 Mar 14];71(8):570-3. Available from: https://europepmc.org/article/med/2369292

[58] Ries AL, Kaplan RM, Myers R, Prewitt LM. Maintenance after pulmonary rehabilitation in chronic lung disease: A randomized trial. Am J Respir Crit Care Med [Internet]. 2003 Mar 15 [cited 2021 Mar 14];167(6):880-8. Available from: https://pubmed.ncbi.nlm.nih.gov/12505859/

[59] Güell R, Casan P, Belda J, Sangenis M, Morante F, Guyatt GH, et al. Long-term effects of outpatient rehabilitation of COPD: A randomized trial. Chest [Internet]. 2000 [cited 2021 Mar 14];117(4):976-83. Available from: https://pubmed.ncbi.nlm.nih.gov/10767227/

[60] Foglio K, Bianchi L, Ambrosino N. Is it really useful to repeat outpatient pulmonary rehabilitation programs in patients with chronic airway obstruction? A 2-year controlled study. Chest [Internet]. 2001 [cited 2021 Mar 14];119(6):1696-704. Available from: https://pubmed.ncbi.nlm.nih.gov/11399693/

[61] Gosselink R. Respiratory rehabilitation: improvement of short- and long-term outcome.

[62] Houchen-Wolloff L, Steiner MC. Pulmonary rehabilitation at a time of

social distancing: Prime time for tele-rehabilitation? [Internet]. Vol. 75, Thorax. BMJ Publishing Group; 2020 [cited 2021 Mar 20]. p. 446-7. Available from: https://www.

[63] Bhatt SP. It's time to rehabilitate pulmonary rehabilitation [Internet]. Vol. 16, Annals of the American Thoracic Society. American Thoracic Society; 2019 [cited 2021 Mar 20]. p. 55-7. Available from: https://www.atsjournals.org/doi/10.1513/AnnalsATS.201809-641ED

[64] Chaplin E, Hewitt S, Apps L, Bankart J, Pulikottil-Jacob R, Boyce S, et al. Interactive web-based pulmonary rehabilitation programme: A randomised controlled feasibility trial. BMJ Open [Internet]. 2017 Mar 1 [cited 2021 Mar 24];7(3):e013682. Available from: http://bmjopen.bmj.com/

[65] Vasilopoulou M, Papaioannou AI, Kaltsakas G, Louvaris Z, Chynkiamis N, Spetsioti S, et al. Home-based maintenance tele-rehabilitation reduces the risk for acute exacerbations of COPD, hospitalisations and emergency department visits. Eur Respir J [Internet]. 2017 May 1 [cited 2021 Mar 24];49(5):1602129. Available from: https://doi.org/10.1183/13993003.02129-2016].

[66] Bhatt SP, Patel SB, Anderson EM, Baugh D, Givens T, Schumann C, et al. Video telehealth pulmonary rehabilitation intervention in chronic obstructive pulmonary disease reduces 30-day readmissions [Internet]. Vol. 200, American Journal of Respiratory and Critical Care Medicine. American Thoracic Society; 2019 [cited 2021 Mar 24]. p. 511-3. Available from: https://www.atsjournals.org/doi/10.1164/rccm.201902-0314LE

[67] Brennan D, Tindall L, Theodoros D, Brown J, Campbell M, Christiana D, et al. A Blueprint for Telerehabilitation Guidelines. Int J Telerehabilitation [Internet]. 2010 Oct 27 [cited 2021 Mar 24];2(2):31-4. Available from: https://telerehab.pitt.edu/ojs/index.php/Telerehab/article/view/6063

[68] Vasilopoulou M, Papaioannou AI, Kaltsakas G, Louvaris Z, Chynkiamis N, Spetsioti S, et al. Home-based maintenance tele-rehabilitation reduces the risk for acute exacerbations of COPD, hospitalisations and emergency department visits. Eur Respir J [Internet]. 2017 May 1 [cited 2021 Mar 20];49(5):1602129. Available from: https://doi.org/10.1183/13993003.02129-2016].

[69] Delivering pulmonary rehabilitation via telehealth during COVID-19 - Communities of practice [Internet]. [cited 2021 Mar 24]. Available from: https://www.health.nsw.gov.au/Infectious/covid-19/communities-of-practice/Pages/guide-pulmonary-rehabilitation.aspx

Chapter 6

Nutritional Status and COPD

Anca Mihaela Hâncu, Florin Mihălțan,
Mihaela Ionela Vladu and Maria Moța

Abstract

Since chronic obstructive pulmonary disease COPD and obesity became global public health challenges, the nutritional status evaluation is more important. How malnutrition and obesity will impact COPD prognosis and treatment is relevant and we considered need a separate approach. The new adiposity based chronic disease concept explains the role played by adiposity, and important studies, like European Community Health Survey ECRHS are highlighting the correlation between adiposity and lung function decline. On the other side, malnutrition decreases effort capacity and impairs the strength of respiratory muscles. Foods, nutrients and dietary patterns are influencing COPD prognosis and Mediterranean Diet, integrated in a healthy lifestyle should be part of COPD management. The important benefic role played by fibers, whole grains, combined with anti-inflammatory and antioxidant effects of fruits and vegetables, together with poly-unsaturated fatty acids PUFA, fish, vitamins and minerals, is detailed below, in contrast with the detrimental role of Western Diet. A multidisciplinary approach in COPD should be considered, integrating lifestyle interventions as important tools in COPD management.

Keywords: obesity, lung function, malnutrition, COPD, nutritional intervention, lifestyle

1. Introduction

Nutritional status and chronic obstructive pulmonary disease COPD.

COPD definition & prevalence. A global public health challenge that can be prevented and treated, COPD is the 4th leading cause of death, estimated to become the 3rd. According to Global Initiative for Chronic Obstructive Lung Disease GOLD 2020, "COPD is a common, preventable and treatable disease that is characterized by persistent respiratory symptoms and airflow limitation that is due to airway and/or alveolar abnormalities usually caused by significant exposure to noxious particles or gases and influenced by host factors including abnormal lung development" [1].

Prevalence- Worldwide, COPD is underdiagnosed and under-recognized, with a medium of <6% of the adult population described in studies. However, most of the studies define COPD by spirometry, not combining symptoms, limiting prevalence description [1].

Nutritional status evaluation. Body mass index BMI (weight per square height) is not the only criteria which defines nutritional status, moreover other measurements, like bioimpedance will describe better the muscle mass, lean mass and adipose tissue. In COPD, the challenge will be to preserve, muscle mass, in order to support lung function. In scientific research dual energy X ray absorptiometry DXA, magnetic resonance imaging MRI are also used to evaluate body composition, but in daily clinical practice, bioimpedance is widely used.

Importance in COPD. Malnutrition, cachexia, obesity represent important co-morbidities, with impact on COPD evolution, treatment and mortality.

2. Obesity

Definition- Adiposity based chronic disease; Abdominal obesity. The concept of cardiometabolic chronic disease, elaborated by Rippe [2] and Mechanick [3] some years ago gain more acceptance. It defines 4 stages: risk, pre-disease, disease and complications for 3 entities: Adiposity based chronic disease ABCD, dysglycemic based chronic disease DBCD, cardiometabolic based chronic disease CMBCD. Practically, instead of obesity, a more complex approach is suggested, named ABCD. The risk stage combines genetics, environment with behavior. The second stage pre-disease describes the increased amount of adipose tissue with abnormal function and distribution. The third stage is classifying obesity based on BMI, with antropometrics and biochemical tests. The fourth stage is defining complications which are cardiometabolic and biomechanical. This more detailed approach is suggesting better the multifactorial interdependence in obesity and the important role played by adiposity.

Prevalence. Worldwide, overweight prevalence is 39% and obesity 13%, meaning 650 mil obese people and 2 bil overweight [4] being an important healthcare issue. In order to better understand the impact of obesity on COPD evolution, analyzing actual studies results is important.

3. Lung function decline and obesity

3.1 European Community Respiratory Health Survey ECRHS

ECRHS is the longest prospective populational study, multicentric that involved 18000 adults along 20 years in 3 phases [5]. Very detailed information have been obtained on forced vital capacity FVC, forced expiratory volume in first second FEV1 as lung function markers. Weight changes were considered as: moderate weight gain 0,25–1 kg/year; stable weight +/– 0,25 kg/year; weight loss –0,25 kg/year. As pulmonary disease diagnosis, asthma was noted. Records about lifestyle were available: smoking status, physical activity, leisure time. Results are summarized below in **Table 1**.

How these data may be interpreted? Weight gain is leading to an accelerated decline of FVC and FEV1, independent of initial weight, normal, overweight or underweight. Clinically, an accelerated decline of pulmonary function was noticed. FEV1/FVC ratio was not altered during weight gain, suggesting the possible restrictive syndrome associated with obesity. For underweight group, surprisingly, FEV1 and FVC decline is attenuated, but the decline of FEV1/FVC ratio is accentuated, concluding that the airflow limitation typical for obstructive pulmonary syndrome may be favorized. Obese people who lost weight during the study period have an attenuated FVC and FEV1 decline suggesting the role played by obesity in the respiratory function and the importance of including obese people in comprehensive lifestyle interventions for restoring a good pulmonary function.

Baseline- young adulthood	Follow- up for 20 years	FVC, FEV1 at the end of the study	FEV1/FVC at the end of the study
Normal BMI, overweight and obese	Increase Weight	FVC and FEV1 accelerated decline	Without decline
Obesity	Decrease Weight	FVC and FEV1 attenuated decline	Without decline
Underweight as teenagers	Stable weight	FVC and FEV1 attenuated decline	FEV1/FVC ratio in an accelerated decline

Adapted after [5].

Table 1.
Conclusions from ECRHS results.

3.2 The Chinese study

A very large Chinese study included 452259 participants with diagnosed COPD, with a follow-up period of 10.1 years [6]. 10739 hospitalization events and deaths have been reported. The study concluded that underweight, with a BMI < 18,5 represents an increased risk of COPD, adjusted hazard ratio HR 1.78 (95% CI, 1.66–1.89). Abdominal obesity was positively associated with COPD risk, after adjustment for BMI. In conclusion, both, abdominal adiposity measures and BMI should be considered for COPD prevention.

3.3 Adipose tissue is not inert, but is acting like an endocrine organ

Adipose tissue may be considered a systemic modulator, influencing the response to environmental exposures and should be considered a potential target for future therapeutic interventions. As an endocrine organ, adipose tissue secretes adipokines, which are adipocyte derived factors that could affect airways function. Not only the inflammatory role recognized for leptin, but the anorexigenic role, accelerated metabolism, modulating immune function together with driving ventilatory regulation will influence pulmonary function [7, 8]. Leptin is supposed to increase bronchial hyperreactivity [9] . In contrast, adiponectin is the anti-inflammatory adipokine, exclusively produced by adipocytes. In lean persons their activity is normal, but decrease in obese patients. Hypoxia, adipose tissue inflammation, macrophage infiltration in adipose tissue will induce finally insulin resistance [9].

3.4 Obesity paradox

Many years ago, in 2002 Gruberg used for the first time the term" obesity paradox" to characterize the lower risk of complications and mortality observed for overweight and obese people versus normal weight or underweight patients in coronary heart disease, pulmonary hypertension, heart failure, stroke, hypertension [10]. Not well elucidated, the concept of obesity paradox is still a subject for study. Increased risk of developing obesity is characterizing patients with COPD, since long term treatment with systemic glucocorticoids is administered [11] and usually a decreased physical activity is seen. Loss of free fat mass FFM, accompanied by muscle weakness and exercise capacity decrease is seen in COPD patients, leading to the conclusion that FFM may be a better predictor than BMI. FFM and weight loss will impact prognosis in COPD [12]. Landbo, Jee [13, 14] described a lower mortality risk for COPD patients with higher BMI. Moreover, Cao [15] described for underweight patients higher risk of mortality compared to leaner counterparts. (HR:0.78; 95% CI:0.65–0.94 and HR:0.69; 95% CI: 0.54–0.89). In this context, the importance of cardiorespiratory fitness CRF should not be neglected. Findings from Aerobic Center Longitudinal Study proved that CRF modify the association between adiposity and results on survival. Fogelholm [16] found a lower all cause/cardiovascular CVD mortality risk for individuals with high BMI and improved aerobic capacity, but this protective effect disappear for BMI > 35 kg/m^2. In a study concluded by Sabino [17] for 32 patients with COPD, higher FFM and exercise capacity lead to better functional outcomes for overweight and obese patients. Practically, obesity paradox is mainly related to CRF and FFM. The role of physical activity PA is well proved in type 2 diabetes, CVD but not well documented in COPD, suggesting potential future correlations and research PA-obesity paradox-CRF and COPD.

In COPD, considering obesity paradox, a question arise: To treat or not to treat? Best strategy is under research, clinicians dilemma is to recommend weight reduction which will improve cardiac performance but may worsen respiratory performance and increase mortality? Which could be the ideal intervention to loose weight? [18].

A new study published in 2020 may propose new answers [19]. The relationship between exacerbation frequency in COPD should be investigated in detail in order to understand better the obesity paradox [20, 21]. This is an observational, retrospective study performed in Netherlands [19] that included 604 patients with COPD, stratified based on BMI level. Lowest five year survival rate was found for underweight and normal weight patients (35%, 41%, p = NS not significant). Survival increased at 47% (p = 0.028) for overweight group, 51% (p = 0.046%) for moderately obese and 63% for severely obese (p = 0.003) patients, versus normal weight patients. Cox regression analysis showed that the effect was independent by other variables and HR = 0.962 (95% CI 0.940–0.984) p = 0.001. The study demonstrated a significant reduction in the exacerbation frequency that required hospitalization in obese patients. Moreover, a significant decrease by 34–40% of readmissions for obese patients was noticed together with a decreased mortality. In contrast with other studies, were the" protective" effect was lost for BMI > 32 kg/m^2, in this study, the group with BMI > 35 kg/m^2 was more protected. The fact that cardiovascular comorbidities, atherosclerosis, is causing a higher mortality rate for leaner patients with COPD should be discussed [22]. Fat reserve, offering a protective source of energy along hospitalization in critical illness should be considered, too. This is supported by better survival rate for critically ill patients with a higher BMI [23, 24]. Preserved muscle mass mean a better prognosis influencing stroke volume and cardiac output [25]. Furthermore, lower systemic vascular resistance is described for obese patients. On the other side, underweight patients, in this study, had an increased mortality, attributed to decreased CRF in the context of lower muscle mass, decreased cardiac output and limited energy storage [23, 24]. Underweight is associated with an increased readmission time in this study, in line with previous data about malnourished patients. How the results of this study should be interpreted? They are limited to specific groups of patients suffering from a disease and should not be considered guidelines for preventive measures at populational level, as authors are mentioning. But, best explanation of this paradox will help the specific approach for future interventions. In conclusion, exacerbation frequency reduction in obese patients with COPD may partially explain obesity paradox, but more prospective research is needed.

4. Malnutrition

4.1 Prevalence

Malnutrition is represented in COPD with a prevalence of 30–60% [26]. Daily energetic expense with respiratory effort is 36–72 kcal/day, normally, but this value may increase by 10 times in COPD. Malnutrition is produced by increased basal metabolic rate, low nutritional intake, or both. The energy spent may be increased more by infections associated with fever.

4.2 The diagnosis of malnutrition

The diagnosis of malnutrition will be based on Global Leadership Initiative on Malnutrition GLIM [27] criteria for the Diagnosis of Malnutrition: a consensus report from the Global Clinical Nutrition Community. There are described 3 phenotypic criteria: low BMI, decrease intake or assimilation of food, unintentional weight loss; and 2 etiologic criteria: disease severity, inflammation and muscle mass decrease. For diagnosis, one etiologic and one phenotypic criteria will be mandatory.

Being an unfavorable prognosis in COPD, malnutrition predispose to infections, lead to weight decrease, decrease effort capacity and the strength of respiratory muscles. Moreover infections decrease surfactant production.

Issues to be addressed in COPD: loss of muscle mass is a strong negative prognosis factor, as has been discussed in previous paragraph and should be addressed by a correct medical nutrition therapy that will be detailed later in this chapter.

5. Lung function and individual foods and nutrients in the context of COPD

5.1 Fibers and whole grains

Larger research focused on wholegrain has been done in relation with cardiovascular disease CVD and cancer [28], but independent benefits have been reported in observational studies on lung function [29, 30] and COPD. Synergic effects of phenolic acids, phytic acid, selenium, vitamin E, essential fatty acids, found in whole grains explain documented benefits on respiratory disease, observed in nonrespiratory diseases, too. Large prospective studies [31] revealed a 40% reduction in the COPD risk after higher fiber intake. Epidemiological data associated fiber intake with lower serum levels of C reactive protein and cytokines (interleukin IL 6, tumoral necrosis factor TNF) and high adiponectine levels, with well-known anti-inflammatory effect. Protective effects are seen mainly for cereal fiber intake in current smokers and ex-smokers, but fruits and vegetable fibers are evidenced, too [31, 32].

5.2 Antioxidant and anti-inflammatory foods - fruits and vegetables

The inflammatory/oxidative pathogenetic implications in COPD, as well as nutritional status and the dietary quality in COPD lead to verify the relations between respiratory effects of antioxidants and anti-inflammatory dietary components. In 2 recent Swedish populational studies, beneficial role of high consumption of fruits and vegetables on long term was reflected in a decreased incidence of COPD, 35% decreased risk in men ($p < 0,0001$) and 37% lower risk for women ($p < 0,0001$) consecutive high consumption of fruits (boths) and vegetables (men). This benefit was mainly obvious in smokers [33, 34]. In conclusion fresh, hard fruits and vegetables provide benefits on lung function decline, COPD symptoms, COPD incidence and mortality. Specific, the protective effect in the men cohort was limited to current smokers or ex-smokers, explained probably by increased antioxidative stress level in smoking. Individual food items observed: apples, pears, peppers, green leafy vegetables [33].

5.3 Vitamins

Limited evidence is reported about any benefit of vitamin D supplementation in COPD progression and immune responses. A conclusion can be drawn, for patients with baseline low level of (OH) D < 25 nmol/L supplementation is beneficial in preventing COPD exacerbations [35]. There are described genetic mutations of vit D binding protein associated with decreased vit D levels linked with a higher risk of COPD [36]. Conflicting results are reported with vit D supplementation but in conclusion they pointed out a benefit for patients with low baseline levels of (OH) D < 25 nmol/L, the active metabolite of vitamin D [37]. The antioxidative effect of vitamin E is revealing promising options for lung function decline associated with age. Well recognized action for vitamin C, which protects lung tissue, focusing on lung function maintenance mediated by vitamin C may lead to a greater success in exploring potential targets in preventing pulmonary diseases [38].

5.4 Minerals

Intake of calcium, phosphorus, potassium, iron and selenium are positively associated with lung function measures (measured by FEV1) based on a case control study published in Japan. 35% reduction of COPD risk is inversely correlated with Calcium intake [39]. An independent positive correlation is found between FEV1 and selenium, calcium, iron and chloride but inverse correlation with sodium and potassium in the general population [40]. Cooper and selenium serum levels are also related to higher lung function in other cross-sectional studies [41]. Through its protective effect against bronchoconstriction and inflammation, Magnesium may play a beneficial role in pulmonary function [42]. Further studies are warranted to prove protective effects of some minerals, explained mainly by antioxidant and anti-inflammatory properties.

5.5 Polyunsaturated fatty acids & fish

Higher intake of ω3-PUFA is related to lower levels of cytokine TNF ($OR = 0.46$, $p = 0.049$) in stable patients with COPD. The same study mentioned the association between a high intake of ω 6-PUFA with high inflammatory markers, for example C reactive protein CRP, interleukin 6, IL6. ($OR = 1.96$ for IL-6, $p = 0.034$; for CRP $OR = 1.95$, $p = 0.039$) [43]. Lower FEV1 after higher consumption of ω6-PUFA was evidenced in a large population based cross sectional study, mainly in smokers, with a higher risk of COPD but without relation to ω3-PUFA [44]. Potential fish benefits in the diet might be obvious within the whole diet, as a recent analysis of two large cohorts is suggesting [45]. 4 servings of fish/week were associated with lower risk of newly diagnosed COPD in 2 large US cohorts. A healthy diet including fish and vegetable sources of ω3-PUFA may be beneficial for COPD, as fish intake could reduce the risk of COPD when plant sources of ω3-PUFA intake is high.

5.6 Foods with negative effects on lung function and COPD

A cross sectional analysis of NHNES [46] associated independently an obstructive pattern in spirometry with increased intake of cured meat but also with newly diagnosed COPD patients, independently of Western dietary pattern or other associations [46, 47]. A more recent large populational study from Sweden confirmed the detrimental effect of processed red meat [48, 49] but not unprocessed. Another reference showed an increased risk of readmission from COPD associated with cured meat intake. A meta-analysis, recently summarized results indicating that higher consumption of red processed meat (more than 75-785 g/week) is leading to a 40% increased risk of COPD [50, 51].

6. Dietary patterns and COPD

In COPD pathogenesis, pollution, genetics, smoking, aging, play a role in developing inflammation, oxidative stress, mucus hypersecretion, antioxidant

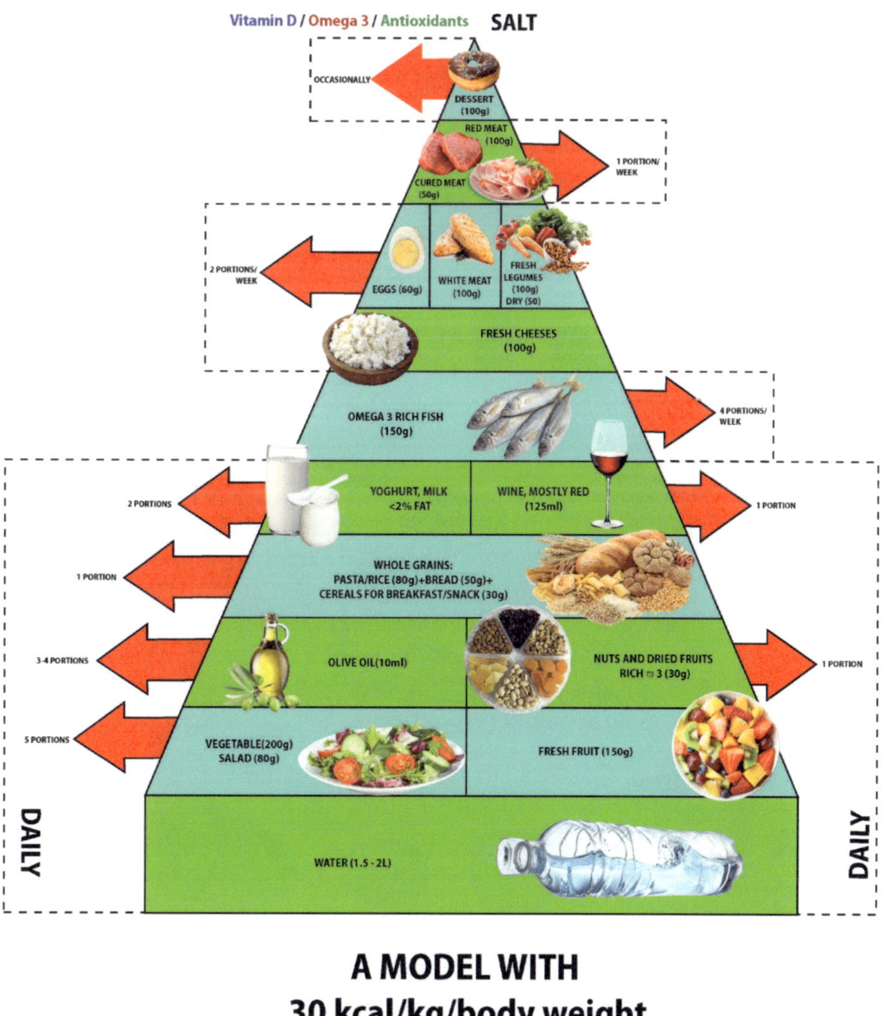

Figure 1.
Food pyramid for subjects with COPD.

depletion, airway remodeling [28] . But lung function is influenced by dietary factors, too. Detrimental role for lung function of Western type diet, characterized by high energy dense food, red and processed food, added sugar, high salt intake, preservatives, low antioxidants, high glycemic index and saturated fats is already proven. By contrast, fruits, vegetables, whole grains, alcohol, wine, legumes, nuts, coffee, fish, high antioxidants, low glycemic index and unsaturated fats, as part of a mediterranean healthy pattern are a support of a healthy lung function. As dietary patterns, is clearly proved the detrimental role of Western model and the protective role of Mediterranean model in COPD.

A special pyramid was designed for COPD patients, represented below, in **Figure 1**, adapted after International Journal of COPD, 2020 [52].

7. Medical nutrition therapy MNT in COPD

Daily energy has to be adapted to activities and requirements calculated by bio-impedance and calorimetry in order to maintain BMI below 30–32 kg/m^2. (special situation in malnutrition is detailed separately). Recommended macronutrients proportion is: 15–25% proteins, 30–45% fats, 40–55% carbohydrates. It has to be underlined that the % of macronutrients is important to maintain (respiratory quotient)RQ, the marker for respiratory tolerance of the pattern recommended. Respiratory quotient, defined as CO_2 volume expired/O_2 volume consumed is the respiratory parameter that indicates food mix metabolized. RQ is 1 for carbohydrates, 0.85 in mixed diets, 0,82 for proteins and 0.7 for fat. The macronutrient percentage is important, correct diet, but not overconsumption will be critical for COPD patients which have compromised ability for gas exchanges, because excess calories produce CO_2 that must be expired and will influence the respiratory process [26]. Considering drug-food interactions, special attention should be considered for salt intake during oral corticosteroid treatment, that should be minimized. Meanwhile, due to increased risk for metabolic disorders, especially high glycaemia, sugar intake should be limited [26].

7.1 MNT in obesity

Muscle mass decrease is a risk factor for mortality from COPD and muscle mass maintenance is important. Considering these, the recommended daily protein intake is 1,2–1,5 g/kgb/day, combined with physical exercises, much more compared to general population recommendations of 0.75–1 g/kgb/day [53]. General recommendations, specified in the 2019 obesity guidelines [54] should be emphasized: decreasing food energetic density, avoid skipping meals, but also snacking, eating just as response to hunger sensations and stop eating when satiety appears, eating slowly and mindfully, as an assumed responsibility, not as a restriction.

7.2 MNT in malnutrition

the objective is to address hypermetabolism in order to prevent weight decrease and lean mass decrease. Practically lean mass/muscular mass maintenance is the key for a good prognosis in COPD [26]. From clinician perspective, MNT should address appetite decrease and improper food intake. Main recommendations are: small meals, frequent, nutritional dense. The main meal should be at the time when the energetic level is the highest. It is recommended to rest before meal. The proper caloric intake will be adjusted in order to maintain a BMI of 20–24 kg/m^2. Availability of food which request minimum time to be prepared, eventually pre-prepared is important. To limit alcohol intake <2 portions/day, 30 g is mandatory.

8. Lifestyle recommendations in COPD

All these nutritional recommendations should be integrated in a healthy lifestyle. Mandatory tobacco cessation, gradual increase in physical activity, according to cardiorespiratory fitness score, optimal sleep and mindfulness, seen as a harmony between mind, body, thoughts and feelings will be beneficial for COPD patients. Despite a great interest in managing COPD, there is a gap in recommendations for physical activity (PA), the most commonly prescribed PA is: walking, cycling, strength training and nonspecific aerobic training. Physical activity PA should be part of lifestyle, may be performed in groups, social or independently. People with COPD should be active until breathless or as per their capacity. Recommended PA durations are ranging from 20 to 45 min/day, depending on guideline. For severe patients, to add short intervals rather than a continuous activity is mentioned. No specific guidelines are mentioning sedentary behaviors. Despite the fact that no specific sleep recommendations are in COPD guidelines, we encourage a referral to a sleep specialist [55].

9. Post-COVID 19

Post COVID 19 pulmonary rehabilitation measures, which start in the hospital for moderate cases, will improve symptoms like dyspnea, anxiety, depression and should continue as part of a healthy lifestyle after recovery, for future. A healthy lifestyle, normalizing body weight by adopting a healthy model adapted to caloric and nutritive requirements daily physical activity and an optimal sleep, mindfulness, will remain key principles for COPD patients after SARS-COV2 infection.

10. Conclusion

New concept of cardiometabolic disease reflects in a more appropriate way the role of adipose tissue in all comorbidities developed in obesity. Lung function decline associated with obesity, as it is revealed by important studies may be an interesting relation to be considered in COPD obese patients. Moreover, malnutrition, with the worst prognosis on COPD development will influence patients management. The importance of a healthy dietary pattern in COPD, designed in the new COPD pyramid are suggesting the strong correlation between foods, nutrients in order to achieve best therapeutical results. Medical nutrition therapy in COPD, based on Mediterranean model, with a high % of proteins, integrated in a healthy lifestyle should be part of COPD management. Nutritional status play an important role in future COPD prognosis and a multidisciplinary team with pneumologist, nutritionist and kinetotherapist should cooperate in order to achieve best long term outcomes.

Author details

Anca Mihaela Hâncu[1*], Florin Mihălțan[2], Mihaela Ionela Vladu[3] and Maria Moța[3]

1 Nutriscience Clinic, Bucharest, Romania

2 "Carol Davila" University of Medicine and Pharmacy, Bucharest, Romania

3 University of Medicine and Pharmacy, Craiova, Romania

*Address all correspondence to: ancahancu@gmail.com

References

[1] www.goldcopd.org/gold-reports

[2] J. Rippe, Lifestyle medicine, 3rd edition, 2019

[3] Jeffrey I. Mechanick, Michael E. Farkouh, Jonathan D. Newman , MPH, W. Timothy Garvey, Cardiometabolic-Based Chronic Disease, Addressing Knowledge and Clinical Practice Gaps, JACC STATE-OF-THE-ART REVIEW, Vol. 7 5, No. 5, 2020, doi.org/10.1016/j.jacc.2019.11.044

[4] Heng He, Bin Wang, Min Zhou, Limin Cao, Weihong Qiu, Ge Mu, Ailian Chen, Shijie Yang, Weihong Chen, Systemic Inflammation Mediates the Associations Between Abdominal Obesity Indices and Lung Function Decline in a Chinese General Population Diabetes, Metabolic Syndrome and Obesity: Targets and Therapy 2020:13 141-150 141, doi.org/10.2147/dmso.s229749

[5] Gabriela P. Peralta GP, et al. (2020). Body mass index and weight change are associated with adult lung function trajectories: the prospective ECRHS study Thorax, dx.doi.org/10.1136/thoraxjnl-2019-213880

[6] Li J, Zhu L, Wei Y, et al. Association between adiposity measures and COPD risk in Chinese adults. Eur Respir J 2020; 55: 1901899, doi.org/10.1183/13993003.01899-2019

[7] Polotsky VY, Smaldone MC, Scharf MT, et al. Impact of interrupted leptin pathways on ventilatory control. J Appl Physiol (1985) 2004 3;96(3):991-8. doi.org/10.1152/japplphysiol.00926.2003

[8] Bassi M, Furuya WI, Menani JV, et al. Leptin into the ventrolateral medulla facilitates chemorespiratory response in leptin-deficient (ob/ob) mice. Acta Physiol (Oxf) 2014 5;211(1):240-8, doi.org/10.1111/apha.12257

[9] Emiel F. M. Wouters, Transatlantic airway conference, Obesity and Metabolic Abnormalities in Chronic Obstructive Pulmonary Disease Department of Respiratory Medicine, Maastricht University Medical Center, Maastricht, the Netherlands, Ann Am Thorac Soc Vol 14, Supplement 5, pp S389–S394, Nov 2017, Copyright © 2017 by the American Thoracic Society, DOI: 10.1513/AnnalsATS.201705-371AW

[10] Prerana Chittal, Abraham Samuel Babu, and Carl J. Lavie. Obesity Paradox: Does Fat Alter Outcomes in Chronic Obstructive Pulmonary Disease? COPD, 00:1-5, 2014, doi.org/10.3109/15412555.2014.915934

[11] Franssen FME, O'Donnell DE, Blaak EE, Schols AMWJ. Obesity and the lung: 5. Obesity and COPD. Thorax 2008; 63:1110-1117. doi.org/10.1136/thx.2007.086827

[12] Jensen LG, Ezzell L. Malnutrition in chronic obstructive pulmonary disease. Am J Clin Nutr 2000; 72:1415-1416 doi.org/10.1093/ajcn/72.6.1415

[13] Landbo C, Prescott E, Lange P, et al. Prognostic value of nutritional status in chronic obstructive pulmonary disease. Am J Respir Crit Care Med 1999; 160:1856-1861. doi.org/10.1164/ajrccm.160.6.9902115

[14] Jee SH, Sull JW, Park J, et al. Body-mass index and mortality in Korean men and women. N Engl J Med 2006; 355:779-787. DOI: 10.1056/NEJMoa054017

[15] Cao C, Wang R, Wang J, Bunjhoo H, Xu Y, Xiong W. Body mass index and mortality in chronic obstructive pulmonary disease: a

meta-analysis. PLoS One. 2012; 7(8):e43892. doi: 10.1371/journal.pone.0043892

[16] M. Fogelholm. Physical activity, fi tness and fatness: relations to mortality, morbidity and disease risk factors. A systematic review. Obesity Rev 2010; 11:202-221. doi.org/10.1111/j.1467-789X.2009.00653.x

[17] Sabino GP, Silva BM, Brunetto AF. Nutritional status is related to fat-free mass, exercise capacity and inspiratory strength in severe chronic obstructive pulmonary disease. Clinics 2010; 65:599-605. doi.org/10.1590/s1807-59322010000600007

[18] Vanessa M Mc Donald, Lisa G Wood, Anne E Holland, Peter Gibson, "Obesity in COPD: To treat or not to treat? " Expert Review of respiratory medicine 2017 vol 11, NO 2, 81-83, doi.org/10.1080/17476348.2017.1267570

[19] Lian Smulders, Anniek van der Aalst, Erik D. E. T. Neuhaus, Sharona Polman, Frits M. E. Franssen; Decreased Risk of COPD Exacerbations in Obese Patients COPD: Journal of Chronic Obstructive Pulmonary Disease: Vol 17, No 5 (tandfonline.com) 2020. doi.org/10.1080/15412555.2020.1799963

[20] Wei YF, Tsai YH, Wang CC, et al. Impact of overweight and obesity on acute exacerbations of COPD - subgroup analysis of the Taiwan Obstructive Lung Disease cohort. Int J Chron Obstruct Pulmon Dis. 2017;12:2723-2729. DOI:10.2147/COPD.S138571

[21] Wu Z, Yang D, Ge Z, et al. Body mass index of patients with chronic obstructive pulmonary disease is associated with pulmonary function and exacerbations: a retrospective real world research. J Thorac Dis. 2018;10(8):5086-5099. DOI:10.21037/jtd. 2018.08.67

[22] Blum A, Simsolo C, Sirchan R, et al. Obesity paradox" in chronic obstructive pulmonary disease. Isr Med Assoc J. 2011;13(11):672-675.

[23] Pepper DJ, Sun J, Welsh J, et al. Increased body mass index and adjusted mortality in ICU patients with sepsis or septic shock: a systematic review and meta-analysis. Crit Care. 2016;20(1):181.DOI:10.1186/s13054-016-1360-z

[24] Zhao Y, Li Z, Yang T, et al. Is body mass index associated with outcomes of mechanically ventilated adult patients in intensive critical units? A systematic review and meta-analysis. PLoS One.2018;13(6):e0198669. DOI:10.1371/journal.pone.0198669

[25] Carbone S, Lavie CJ, Arena R. Obesity and heart failure: focus on the obesity paradox. Mayo Clin Proc. 2017;92(2):266-279. DOI:10.1016/j.mayocp.2016.11.001

[26] L Kathleen Mahan, Janice L Raymond, "Krause's Food and Nutrition care process" 2020, 15th edition, 689

[27] Gordon L. Jensen, MD, GLIM Criteria for the Diagnosis of Malnutrition: A Consensus Report From the Global Clinical Nutrition Community. Journal of Parenteral and Enteral Nutrition Volume 43 Number 1 January 2019 32-40, 2018 Elsevier Ltd, the European Society for Clinical Nutrition and Metabolism and American Society for Parenteral and Enteral Nutrition. All rights reserved DOI: 10.1002/jpen.1440 wileyonlinelibrary.com

[28] Egeria Scoditti, Marika Massaro, Sergio Garbarino and Domenico Maurizio Toraldo, Role of Diet in Chronic Obstructive Pulmonary Disease Prevention and Treatment Nutrients 2019, 11, 1357; doi:10.3390/nu11061357

[29] Tabak, C.; Smit, H.A.; Heederik, D.; Ocke, M.C.; Kromhout, D. Diet and chronic obstructive pulmonary

disease: Independent beneficial effects of fruits, whole grains, and alcohol (the MORGEN study). Clin. Exp.Allergy 2001, 31, 747-755. doi: 10.1046/j.1365-2222.2001.01064.x.

[30] Root, M.M.; Houser, S.M.; Anderson, J.J.; Dawson, H.R. Healthy Eating Index 2005 and selected macronutrients are correlated with improved lung function in humans. Nutr. Res. 2014, 34, 277-284. doi.org/10.1016/j.nutres.2014.02.008

[31] Kaluza, J.; Harris, H.; Wallin, A.; Linden, A.; Wolk, A. Dietary Fiber Intake and Risk of Chronic Obstructive Pulmonary Disease: A Prospective Cohort Study of Men. Epidemiology 2018, 29, 254-260. doi: 10.1097/EDE.0000000000000750.

[32] Varraso, R.;Willett,W.C.; Camargo, C.A., Jr. Prospective study of dietary fiber and risk of chronic obstructive pulmonary disease among US women and men. Am. J. Epidemiol. 2010, 171, 776-784. doi: 10.1093/aje/kwp455. Epub 2010 Feb 19.

[33] Kaluza, J.; Larsson, S.C.; Orsini, N.; Linden, A.; Wolk, A. Fruit and vegetable consumption and risk of COPD: A prospective cohort study of men. Thorax 2017, 72, 500-509. doi: 10.1136/thoraxjnl-2015-207851. Epub 2017 Feb 22.

[34] Kaluza, J.; Harris, H.R.; Linden, A.; Wolk, A. Long-term consumption of fruits and vegetables and risk of chronic obstructive pulmonary disease: A prospective cohort study of women. Int. J. Epidemiol. 2018, 47, 1897-1909. doi.org/10.1093/ije/dyy178

[35] Jolli_e, D.A.; Greenberg, L.; Hooper, R.L.; Mathyssen, C.; Rafiq, R.; de Jongh, R.T.; Camargo, C.A.; Gri_ths, C.J.; Janssens, W.; Martineau, A.R.; et al. Vitamin D to prevent exacerbations of COPD: Systematic review and meta-analysis of individual participant data from randomised controlled trials. Thorax 2019, 74, 337-345. doi.org/10.1136/bmj.l1025

[36] Janssens, W.; Bouillon, R.; Claes, B.; Carremans, C.; Lehouck, A.; Buysschaert, I.; Coolen, J.; Mathieu, C.; Decramer, M.; Lambrechts, D.; et al. Vitamin D deficiency is highly prevalent in COPD and correlates with variants in the vitamin D-binding gene. Thorax 2010, 65, 215-220. doi: 10.1136/thx.2009.120659. Epub 2009 Dec 8.

[37] Jollie, D.A.; Greenberg, L.; Hooper, R.L.; Mathyssen, C.; Rafiq, R.; de Jongh, R.T.; Camargo, C.A.; Griths, C.J.; Janssens, W.; Martineau, A.R. et al. Vitamin D to prevent exacerbations of COPD: Systematic review and of individual participant data from randomised controlled trials. Thorax 2019, 74, doi.org/10.1136/thoraxjnl-2018-212092

[38] Ting Zhai, Shizhen Li, Wei Hei, Potential micronutrients and phytochemicals against the pathogenesis of COPD and lung cancer, Nutrients, 2018. 337-345. doi.org/10.3390/nu10070813

[39] Hirayama, F.; Lee, A.H.; Oura, A.; Mori, M.; Hiramatsu, N.; Taniguchi, H. Dietary intake of six minerals in relation to the risk of chronic obstructive pulmonary disease. Asia Pac. J. Clin. Nutr. 2010, 19, 572-577.

[40] McKeever, T.M.; Lewis, S.A.; Smit, H.A.; Burney, P.; Cassano, P.A.; Britton, J. A multivariate analysis of serum nutrient levels and lung function. Respir. Res. 2008, 9, 67. DOI: 10.1186/1465-9921-9-67

[41] Pearson, P.; Britton, J.; McKeever, T.; Lewis, S.A.; Weiss, S.; Pavord, I.; Fogarty, A. Lung function and blood levels of copper, selenium, vitamin C and vitamin E in the general population. Eur. J. Clin. Nutr. 2005, 59, 1043-1048. doi.org/10.1038/sj.ejcn.1602209

[42] Al Alawi, A.M.; Majoni, S.W.; Falhammar, H. Magnesium and Human Health: Perspectives and Research Directions. Int. J. Endocrinol. 2018, 9041694 dx.doi.org/10.1155%2F2018%2F9041694

[43] de Batlle, J.; Sauleda, J.; Balcells, E.; Gomez, F.P.; Mendez, M.; Rodriguez, E.; Barreiro, E.; Ferrer, J.J.; Romieu, I.; Gea, J.; et al. Association between Omega3 and Omega6 fatty acid intakes and serum inflammatory markers in COPD. J. Nutr. Biochem. 2012, 23, 817-821 .doi.org/10.1016/j.jnutbio.2011.04.005

[44] McKeever, T.M.; Lewis, S.A.; Cassano, P.A.; Ocke, M.; Burney, P.; Britton, J.; Smit, H.A. The relation between dietary intake of individual fatty acids, FEV1 and respiratory disease in Dutch adults. Thorax 2008, 63, 208-214. doi.org/10.1136/thx.2007.090399

[45] Varraso, R.; Barr, R.G.;Willett,W.C.; Speizer, F.E.; Camargo, C.A., Jr. Fish intake and risk of chronic obstructive pulmonary disease in 2 large US cohorts. Am. J. Clin. Nutr. 2015, 101, 354-361. doi.org/10.3945/ajcn.114.094516

[46] Jiang, R.; Paik, D.C.; Hankinson, J.L.; Barr, R.G. Cured meat consumption, lung function, and chronic obstructive pulmonary disease among United States adults. Am. J. Respir. Crit. Care Med. 2007, 175. DOI: 10.1164/rccm.200607-969OC

[47] Varraso, R.; Jiang, R.; Barr, R.G.; Willett, W.C.; Camargo, C.A., Jr. Prospective study of cured meats consumption and risk of chronic obstructive pulmonary disease in men. Am. J. Epidemiol. 2007, 166, doi.org/10.1093/aje/kwm235

[48] Jiang, R.; Camargo, C.A., Jr.; Varraso, R.; Paik, D.C.; Willett,W.C.; Barr, R.G. Consumption of cured meats and prospective risk of chronic obstructive pulmonary disease in women. Am. J. Clin. Nutr. 2008, 87, 1002-1008. doi.org/10.1093/ajcn/87.4.1002

[49] Kaluza, J.; Larsson, S.C.; Linden, A.; Wolk, A. Consumption of Unprocessed and Processed Red Meat and the Risk of Chronic Obstructive Pulmonary Disease: A Prospective Cohort Study of Men. Am. J. Epidemiol. 2016, 184, 829-836 .doi.org/10.1093/aje/kww101

[50] de Batlle, J.; Mendez, M.; Romieu, I.; Balcells, E.; Benet, M.; Donaire-Gonzalez, D.; Ferrer, J.J.; Orozco-Levi, M.; Anto, J.M.; Garcia-Aymerich, J.; et al. Cured meat consumption increases risk of readmission in COPD patients. Eur. Respir. J. 2012, 40, 555-560 .doi.org/10.1183/09031936.00116911

[51] Salari-Moghaddam, A.; Milajerdi, A.; Larijani, B.; Esmaillzadeh, A. Processed red meat intake and risk of COPD: A systematic review and dose-response meta-analysis of prospective cohort studies. Clin. Nutr. 2018, 38, 1109-1116 .doi.org/10.1016/j.clnu.2018.05.020

[52] Mariangela Rondanelli, Milena Anna Faliva, Gabriella Peroni, Vittoria Infantino, Clara Gasparri, Giancarlo Iannello, Simone Perna, Tariq AbdulKarim Alalwan, Salwa Al-Thawadi, Angelo Guido, CorsicoFood, Pyramid for Subjects with Chronic Obstructive Pulmonary Diseases, International Journal of Chronic Obstructive Pulmonary Disease, 2020:15 1435-1448

[53] Rebecca F. Mc Loughlin, Vanessa M. McDonald, Peter G. Gibson, Hayley A. Scott, Michael J. Hensley, Lesley MacDonald-Wicks and Lisa G. Wood, The Impact of a Weight Loss Intervention on Diet Quality and Eating Behaviours in People with Obesity and COPD, Nutrients, 2017 Oct 20;9(10):1147. doi.org/10.3390/nu9101147

[54] Durrer Schutz et al, "Management of obesity by GP's" Obesity Facts 2019; 12;40-66, doi.org/10.1159/000496183

[55] Hayley Lewthwaite, Tanja W Effing, Timothy Olds and Maric T Williams, Physical activity, sedentary behaviour and sleep in COPD guidelines: A systematic review, Chronic Respiratory Disease 2017, Vol. 14(3) 231-244. doi.org/10.1177%2F1479972316687224

Chapter 7

Mechanical Ventilation for Patients with COPD

Ozlem Ediboglu

Abstract

Mechanical ventilation is a lifesaving therapy in patients who have acute respiratory failure due to chronic obstructive pulmonary disease (COPD). Mechanical ventilaton either invasive or non-invasive has an important role in the management of acute exacerbation of COPD (AECOPD). AECOPD required hospitalizaton had increased mortality and poor prognosis. Ventilatory management success related to understanding physiopathology of the disease. Clinicians must be aware of deterioration of clinical signs of COPD patients. The most appropriate treatment should be performed at optimal time. Some COPD patients are at high risk for prolonged mechanical ventilation due to COPD is a progressive disease.

Keywords: mechanical ventilation, COPD, respiratory failure

1. Introduction

Chronic obstructive pulmonary disease (COPD) is a major global health problem which has high morbidity and mortality [1]. COPD is characterized by chronic inflammation of the airways and lung parenchyma. The most important physiologic abnormality is worsening of expiratory airflow limitation due to increased airway resistance and decreased elastic recoil [2]. Patients who have fexpiratory airflow limitation cannot breath normally and due to dynamic hyperinflation increase work of breathing. These physiologic changes are deteriorated unless avoid risk factors because of COPD is a progressive disease and can be complicated with different severity of acute exacerbation [1–4].

Acute exacerbation of chronic obstructive pulmonary disease (AECOPD) is described an acute worsening of the clinical condition of the COPD patient [5]. Clinical features are highly variable and AECOPD has a negative impact of patients' health status and outcomes [1, 6–8]. The reported mortality associated with a AECOPD is variably at 11% to 32% [9]. The mortality rate and costs are much higher in some patients requiring mechanical ventilation [10, 11]. In severe AECOPD, it is crucial to recognise acute respiratory failure (ARF) immediately and to decide appropriate treatment. ARF is defined as the inability to maintain the delivery of oxygen and/or removal of carbon dioxide acutely. Worsening gas exchange and consequently hypercapnia and/or hypoxemia occur in arterial blood gas sample (ABG) analysis [12].

2. Non-invasive ventilation

Mechanical ventilation either invasive or non- invasive is lifesaving treatment for acute respiratory failure. It is targeted by non - invasive ventilation (NIV)

to minimize risks of mechanical ventilation and maximize patients' safety and comfort. Hence NIV is successful to provide alveolar ventilation and gas exchange as invasive mechanical ventilation (IMV); NIV accepted widely as the first choice in treating AECOPD patients with ARF [13–24]. NIV therapy success is related to appropriate patient selection and early application [14, 25–27]. The appropriate patient means that is alert, co-operative, compliant and has no contraindications [28].

NIV is applied after initial treatment if the pH remains <7.30 and after exclusion of reversible precipitating causes such as a pneumothorax, the depressant effect of uncontrolled oxygen therapy, or the excessive use of sedatives [29–31]. According to GOLD guide, NIV is considered at least one of these conditions; respiratory acidosis, weakness of respiratory muscles, severe dyspnea, increased work of breathing, accessory muscle using, intercostal retraction, paradoxal breathing and persistant hypoxemia with oxygen therapy [32]. Main determinants are experience of the clinician, place of the NIV therapy, clinical condition and theurapeutic requirement of patient [33, 34].

NIV can be apply with all ventilators used in IMV support [35]. It's important to known technical specialities and settings by clinician. Portable ventilators, intermediate ventilators and ICU ventilators has been used [33, 36]. Portable ventilators are named according to targeted parameter as volume and pressure ventilators. The synonim name is portable device is bilevel or BiPAP (Bilevel positive airway pressure) ventilator. Clinicians must be aware of difference between settings of the two devices: While adjusting IPAP (inspiratory positive airway pressure), EPAP (expiratory positive airway pressure) levels setting in BiPAP device, pressure support (PS = IPAP - EPAP) and EPAP levels in ICU ventilators [33, 37]. Bi-level pressure support ventilators are simpler to use, cheaper, and more flexible than other types of ventilator currently available. ICU ventilators have full monitoring and alarm capability and can be given up to 100% FiO_2 when needed [30, 33]. Whole appropriate equipment must be ready to iniciate the NIV therapy as single/double lumen circuit, nasal/oronasal NIV mask by different size [38]. Mask selection is more important than ventilator. In acute setting, oronasal mask is well tolerated and preferred by many clinicians [14, 38, 39].

NIV is contraindicated in these situations; respiratory or cardiac arrest, hemodynamic instability, inability to use mask, excessive secretion, high risk for aspiration, and uncooperative patient.

Initially it is began with low pressure levels as IPAP 8–10 cm H_2O and EPAP 4–5 cm H_2O. According to patient's clinical status, pressure levels can be increased. Monitorization of clinical signs, parameters of mechanical ventilation and gas exchange at the bedside are very important. Especially clinician must be follow and record subjective symptoms like anxiety, consciousness, delirium, agitation, sedation, analgesia, patient comfort, dyspnea, tolerance of mask. All the time NIV therapy, physiological response like respiratory rate (RR), using accessory muscle, heart rate (HR) and rhythm, blood pressure (BP) must be recorded. After the first 1–2 hours ABG must be done. We must consider intubation, if no improvement in ABG, deterioration in level of consciousness, NIV poorly tolerated, and inadequate secretion clearance [1, 7, 21, 40].

NIV failure is associated with hospital mortality, length of hospital and ICU stay [41]. NIV failure indicators are found as initial pH <7.25, Glascow Coma Scale (GCS) <10, Acute Physiology and Chronic Health Evaluation (APACHE) II score > 25, severe comorbidity, asynchrony, leaks [7, 42], existing pneumonia, and bad initial response (no change RR, pH and $paCO_2$) [14, 43]. The potential causes NIV failure are defined that poor patient selection, progression of the underlying disease, wrong interface, wrong ventilator, inappropriate ventilator settings and clinican's inexperience [44]. In a study, HACOR scores (heart rate, acidosis, consciousness, oxygenation, respiratory rate) be defined as a potential tool for clinical physicians to identify NIV failure earlier [45]. Patient tolerance to NIV is a critical factor determining its success in avoiding endotracheal intubation [46]. The most important point of the tolerance to NIV is optimal synchrony between the patient's spontaneous breathing activity and the ventilator's set parameters, known as "patient–ventilator interaction" [47]. Clinician can detected an asynchrony index (AI) (%) via visual inspection of asynchrony events (ineffective triggering, auto-triggering, premature cycling, double triggering and delayed cycling). AI is identified as number of asynchrony events/total RR X 100% and above 10% was accepted as severe asynchrony [44]. In a multicenter study, severe asynchrony was found 43% [48]. The level of pressure support and the existing of leaks were found independent predictive factors of severe asynchronies and severe asynchronies were detected 30% of patients [49]. Patient-ventilator synchrony is related to better success of NIV. For this reason, in case of asynchrony, the most appropriate strategies should be followed to improve synchronization with NIV [44].

3. Invasive mechanical ventilation

Endotracheal intubation should be done any one of the following criteria immediately: respiratory arrest, loss of consciousness, psychomotor agitation requiring sedation, hemodynamic instability with a systolic BP less than 70 or greater than 180 mmHg, HR less than 50 beats/minute with loss of alertness, gasping for air. These criteria are named major criteria. Intubation was suggested any two of the following criteria also named minor criteria; RR >35 breath/min, worsening acidemia or pH < 7.25, paO_2 < 40 mmHg or paO_2/FiO_2 < 200 despite oxygen therapy, decreasing level of consciousness [50]. Before intubation preoxygenation is essential. Intubation with the rapid sequence induction and cricoid pressure to reduce the risk of aspiration should ideally be performed by an experienced clinician [51].

After intubation, its targeted to improve gas exchange abnormality and to avoid auto-PEEP ($PEEP_i$) [7, 52]. Dynamic hyperinflation(DHI) may exist before intubation or induced by mechanical ventilation. The minute volume (MV) should be adjusted to pH and not to the $PaCO_2$ levels. Clinicians should be avoid overventilation and $paCO_2$ levels should decreased gradually. It is important to provide lower MV (RR x tidal volume (TV)) and higher inspiratory flow rate which has allow longer expiratory time. Any mode can be used, either assist control (AC), synchronized intermittent mandatory ventilation with either volume or pressure target (SIMV-VS, SIMV-PS), or pressure support ventilation(PSV). Clinician's experience is the most important determinant of mode selection. Initial ventilator settings are recommended like that; TV: 6–10 ml/kg, FiO_2: 1.0, RR: 10–14 breaths/minute, no PEEP, inspiratory flow rate: 80–100 liter/minute with square waveform [1, 2, 4]. Monitoring the lung mechanics on ventilator graphic screen continously and detecting any sign of DHI or $PEEP_i$ are very important. The clinicians should be followed existing any clinical signs to avoid the complications of DHI. The most important complications of DHI are hypotension, hemodynamic collaps, barotrauma and increased work of breathing (WOB) [51, 53]. Therefore, that strategies must be applied by clinicians to reduce auto-PEEP; providing the longest expiratory phase that is possible, reducing patient ventilatory demand and MV, and reducing airflow resistance by bronchodilators and steroids [1].

Barotrauma is an important risk at the COPD patients. Elevated peak inspiratory pressure (PIP) does not reflect the alveolar pressure in patients with bronchospasm.

Alveolar pressure can be detected with plateau pressure (P_{plat}) and suggested PIP < 50 cmH_2O, P_{plat} < 30 cmH_2O to avoid barotrauma [1].

Quantifying $PEEP_i$ is a difficult and favored process. $PEEP_i$ amount of proportionated with degree of bronchial obstruction. Different techniques can be used to calculate $PEEP_i$. Clinicians can directly measure by occluding the expiratory port for 1–3 seconds at end expiration or by using expiratory hold maneuver on new ventilators. Static $PEEP_i$ can be measured in this way only in sedatized patients without active respiratory effort. The $PEEP_i$ can then be calculated by subtracting the external PEEP from the total PEEP. If there is spontan respiratory effort of the patient, dynamic $PEEP_i$ can be determined by simultanously recording esophageal pressure and airflow tracings. It is measured at end expiration as the negative deflection of esophageal pressure to the point of zero flow. The dynamic $PEEP_i$ is usually measured lower than static $PEEP_i$ by reason of different longer of time constant [1, 2, 4, 53, 54]. While $PEEP_i$ is determined extrinsic PEEP ($PEEP_e$) at 80% of $PEEP_i$ should be added to reduce patient triggering effort. Ventilator trigger sensitivity must be justify minimal [1, 4, 6, 51, 55, 56].

Weaning should begin once the cause of the exacerbation is adequately treated and the patient is hemodynamically stable. Physiologic parameters must be followed intensively. It's targeted MV < 15 L, RR < 30 breaths/minute, TV > 325 ml, rapid shallow breathing index (RSBI) <105, maximum inspiratory pressure (MIP) < −15. Although the superiority did not found among each other, different strategies were used to weaning. Daily spontaneous breathing trail (SBT) is one way of identifying patients stable to wean and it may reduce the number of ICU days. While decreasing gradually of PS has not been shown to be superior to SBT, PSV is preferable by many clinicians. Using NIV to facilitate weaning is accepted by multiple RCT [14, 15, 52, 57, 58].

4. High flow oxygen therapy

Long term oxygen therapy (LTOT), is used mainly in COPD patients with chronic hypoxemia [32]. High flow oxygen therapy (HFOT) is a new technique for delivering oxygen. There are many studies using HFOT instead of conventional oxygen therapy (COT) recently. HFOT was well tolerated and was sensed as comfortable. By using this system, oxygen delivery trends provided to be lower, and $paCO_2$ levels could be measured significant decreased. HFOT could be accepted as an alternative treatment to NIV due to it generates a modest degree of positive pressure almost 5–6 cmH_2O. It provides a more physiological humidification and heating of the airways. In this settings, HFOT has been used with different aims, as an alternative to COT, and NIV [59–62].

Author details

Ozlem Ediboglu
University of Health Sciences, Dr Suat Seren Chest Diseases and Surgery Training and Research Hospital, Intensive Care Unit, Izmir, Turkey

*Address all correspondence to: ozlemediboglu@gmail.com

References

[1] Reddy RM, Guntupalli KK. Review of ventilatory techniques to optimize mechanical ventilation in acute exacerbation of chronic obstructive pulmonary disease. Int J COPD 2007;2(4):441-452

[2] Mowery NT. Ventilator Strategies for Chronic Obstructive Pulmonary Disease and Acute Respiratory Syndrome. Surg Clin N Am 2017;97:1381-1397

[3] Levi MO. Structure and function of the respiratory muscles in patients with COPD: impairment or adaptation? Eur Respir J 2003; 22(Suppl 46):41-51s

[4] Ediboglu O. Hasta Tiplerine Gore Mekanik Ventilasyon. Ed. Kunter E, Kıraklı C, Koşar F. Mekanik Ventilasyon. S: 75-89, TÜSAD Eğitim Kitapları Serisi, Probiz Ltd Şti, İstanbul 2013

[5] Vogelmeier CF, Criner GJ, Martinez FJ, et al. Global strategy for the diagnosis, management, and prevention of chronic obstructive lung disease 2017 report: gold executive summary. Eur Respir J 2017; **49**: 1700214

[6] O'Donnell DE, Hernandez P, Kaplan A, et al. Canadian Thoracic Society recommendations for management of chronic obstructive pulmonary disease - 2008 update - highlights for primary care. Can Respir J 2008;15 Suppl A:1A-8A

[7] Kosar F. Kronik Obstruktif Akciğer Hastalığında Akut Solunum Yetmezliği ve Mekanik Ventilasyon. Turk Klin J Pulm Med Spec Topics 2010; 3 (2): 20-28

[8] Ambrosino N, Simonds A. The clinical management in extremely severe COPD. Respir Med 2007; 101 (8):1613-24

[9] Gadre SK, Duggal A, Mireles-Cabodevila E, et al. Acute respiratory failure requiring mechanical ventilation in severe chronic obstructive pulmonary disease (COPD). Medicine (2018) 97:17 (e0487)

[10] Alaithan AM, Memon JI, Rehmani RS, et al. Chronic obstructive pulmonary disease: hospital and intensive care unit outcomes in the Kingdom of Saudi Arabia. Int J Chron Obstruct Pulmon Dis 2012;7:819-823

[11] Raurich JM, Perez J, Ibanez J, et al. In-hospital and 2-year survival of patients treated with mechanical ventilation for acute exacerbation of COPD. Arch Bronconeumol 2004;40:295-300

[12] Breen D, Churches T, Hawker F, et al. Acute respiratory failure secondary to chronic obstructive pulmonary disease treated in the intensive care unit: a long term follow up study. Thorax 2002;57:29-33

[13] Rochwerg B, Brochard L, Elliott MW, Hess D, et al. Official ERS/ATS clinical practice guidelines: noninvasive ventilation for acute respiratory failure. Eur Respir J 2017; 50: 1602426

[14] Lieshhing T, Kwok H, Hill N. Acute applications of noninvasive positive pressure ventilation. Chest 2003:124; 699-713

[15] Garpestad E, Brennan J, Hill N. Noninvasive ventilation for critical care. Chest 2007;132: 711-720

[16] Scala R, Pisani L. Noninvasive ventilation in acute respiratory failure: which recipe for success? Eur Respir Rev 2018;27:180029

[17] Hess D. Noninvasive ventilation for acute respiratory failure. Respir Care 2013;58(6):950-969

[18] Evans TW. International Consensus Conferences in Intensive Care Medicine: noninvasive positive pressure ventilation in acute respiratory failure. Organised jointly by the American Thoracic Society, the European Respiratory Society, the 1394 Mowery European Society of Intensive Care Medicine, and the Societe de Reanimation de Langue Francaise, and approved by the ATS Board of Directors, December 2000. Intensive Care Med 2001;27(1):166-178

[19] Girou E, Brun-Buisson C, Taillé S, et al. Secular trends in nosocomial infections and mortality associated with noninvasive ventilation in patients with exacerbation of COPD and pulmonary edema. JAMA 2003;290(22):2985-2991

[20] Scala R, Naldi M. Ventilators for Noninvasive Ventilation to Treat Acute Respiratory Failure. Respir Care 2008;53(8):1054-1080

[21] Brochard L. Mechanical ventilation: invasive versus noninvasive. Eur Respir J 2003;22: Suppl. 47. 31s–37s

[22] International Consensus Conferences in Intensive Care Medicine: Noninvasive Positive Pressure Ventilation in Acute Respiratory Failure. Am J Respir Crit Care Med. 2001; 163: 283-291

[23] Crimi C, Noto A. A European Survey of Noninvasive Ventilation Practices. Eur Respir J 2010;36:362-369

[24] Schönhofer B, Sortor-Leger S. Equipment needs for noninvasive mechanical ventilation. Eur Respir J 2002;20:1029-1036

[25] Plant PK, Owen JL, Elliott MW. Non-invasive ventilation in acute exacerbations of chronic obstructive pulmonary disease: long term survival and predictors of in-hospital outcome. Thorax 2001;56:708-712

[26] Celikel T, Sungur M, Ceyhan B, et al. Comparison of noninvasive positive pressure ventilation with standard medical therapy in hypercapnic acute respiratory failure. Chest 1998; 114: 1636-1642

[27] Yıldırım F. Kronik Obstrüktif Akciğer Hastalığı Akut Alevlenmede Noninvaziv Mekanik Ventilasyon Kullanımı. Noninvazif Mekanik Ventilasyon Uygulamaları. Ed Ocal S. TÜSAD Eğitim Kitapları Serisi Ekim 2017:119-127

[28] Scala R, Naldi M, Archinucci I, et al. Noninvasive positive pressure ventilation in patients with acute exacerbations of COPD and varying levels of consciousness. Chest 2005; 128(3): 1657-1666

[29] Plant P, Owen J, Elliott M. A multi centre randomised control trial of the early use of non invasive ventilation for acute exacerbations of chronic obstructive pulmonary disease. Lancet 2000;355:1931-1935

[30] British Thoracic Society Standards of Care Subcommittee. Non-invasive ventilation in acute respiratory failure. Thorax 2002;57:192-211

[31] Brochard L. Non invasive ventilation for acute exacerbations of COPD: a new standard of care. Thorax 2000;55:817-818

[32] Global Strategy for the Diagnosis, Management, and Prevention of Chronic Obstructive Pulmonary Disease GOLD 2019 Report

[33] Ediboglu O. Noninvazif Mekanik Ventilasyonda Cihazlar, Noninvazif Mekanik Ventilasyonda Modlar. Z. Karakurt (Ed) Organizasyondan Tedaviye Yoğun Bakım. Türk Toraks Derneği Toraks Kitapları Bölüm 6, 7, 2014

[34] Penuelas O, Frutos Vivar F, Esteban A. Noninvasive positive

pressure ventilation in acute respiratory failure. CMAJ 2007;177(10):1211-1218

[35] Hess DR. The Evidence for Noninvasive Positive-Pressure Ventilation in the Care of Patients in Acute Respiratory Failure. A Systematic Review of the Literature. Respir Care 2004;49(7):810-829

[36] Scala R, Naldi M. Ventilators for Noninvasive Ventilation to Treat Acute Respiratory Failure. Respir Care 2008;53(8):1054-1080

[37] Kaya A, Ciledag A. Yoğun Bakım Ventilatörü ve BiPAP İle Noninvaziv Mekanik Ventilasyon Uygulamalarındaki Farklılıklar. Noninvazif Mekanik Ventilasyon Uygulamaları. Ed Ocal S. TÜSAD Eğitim Kitapları Serisi Ekim 2017

[38] Navalesi P, Fanfulla F, Frigerio P, et al. Physiologic evaluation of noninvasive mechanical ventilation delivered with three types of masks in patients with chronic hypercapnic respiratory failure. Crit Care Med 2000; 28:1785-1790

[39] Uğurlu AO, Ergan B, Takır HB, İn E, Ozyılmaz E, Edipoğlu O,et al. Approach of pulmonologists in Turkey to noninvasive mechanical ventilation use in acute respiratory failure. Tuberk Toraks 2015;63(4):213-225

[40] Ediboglu O. Yoğun Bakımda Akut Solunum Yetmezliği Olan Hastanın Değerlendirilmesi ve Tedavi İlkeleri. Yoğun Bakim Protokolleri. N. Şenoğlu (Ed). Tepecik Hastanesi Yayınları/2017, İzmir

[41] Shah NM, D'Cruz RF, Murphy PB. Update: non-invasive ventilation in chronic obstructive pulmonary disease. T Thorac Dis 2018;10(Suppl 1):S71-S79

[42] Yıldırım F. Noninvaziv Mekanik Ventilasyon Başarısını Etkileyen Fizyolojik Parametreler. Noninvazif Mekanik Ventilasyon Uygulamaları. Ed Ocal S. TÜSAD Eğitim Kitapları Serisi Ekim 2017:28-38

[43] Soo Hoo GW, Santiago S, Williams AJ. Nasal mechanical ventilation for hypercapnic respiratory failure in chronic obstructive pulmonary disease: determinants of success and failure. Crit Care Med 1994; 22:1253-1261

[44] Hess DR. Patient-ventilator interaction during noninvasive ventilation. Respir Care 2011;56(2):153-165

[45] Duan J, Wang S, Liu P, et al. Early prediction of noninvasive ventilation failure in COPD patients: derivation, internal validation, and external validation of a simple risk score. Ann. Intensive Care 2019; 9:108

[46] Carlucci A, Richard J, Wysocki M, et al. Noninvasive versus conventional mechanical ventilation. An epidemiologic survey. Am J Respir Crit Care Med 2001; 163:874-880

[47] Tobin M, Jubran A, Laghi F. Patient-ventilator interaction. Am J Respir Crit Care Med 2001; 163:1059-1063

[48] Vignaux L, Vargas F, Roeseler J, et al. Patient–ventilator asynchrony during non-invasive ventilation for acute respiratory failure: a multicenter study. Intensive Care Med 2009; 35: 840-846

[49] Carlucci A, Pisani L, Malovini A, Nava S. Patient- ventilator asynchronies: may the respiratory mechanics play a role? Crit Care 2013; 17: R54

[50] Brochard L, Mancebo J, Wysocki M, et al. Noninvasive ventilation for acute exacerbations of chronic obstructive pulmonary disease. N Engl J Med 1995; 333(13): 817-822

[51] Blanch L, Bernabe F. Measurement of air trapping, Intrinsic Positive End

Expiratory Pressure and Dynamic Hyperinflation in Mechanically Ventilated Patients. Respir Care 2005;50(1):110-123

[52] Gladwin MT, Pierson DJ. Mechanical ventilation of the patient with severe chronic obstructive pulmonary disease. Intensive Care Med (1998) 24:898-910

[53] Davidson AC. The pulmonary physician in critical care. Critical care management of respiratory failure resulting from COPD. Thorax 2002;57:1079-1084

[54] Ward NS, Dushay KM. Clinical concise review: Mechanical ventilation of patients with chronic obstructive pulmonary disease. Crit Care Med 2008 Vol. 36, No. 5: 1614-1619

[55] Köhnlein T, Welte T. Ventilation in Obstructive Lung Disease Chapter 3. Eur Respir Mon 2006;36:34-48

[56] Guerin C, Milic-Emili J, Fournier G: Effect of PEEP on work of breathing in mechanically ventilated COPD patients. Intensive Care Med 2000; 26:1207-1214

[57] Esteban A, Frutos F, Tobin NJ, et al. A comparison of four methods of weaning patients from mechanical ventilation. N Eng J Med 1995; 332:345

[58] Brochard L, Rauss A, Benito S, et al. Comparison of three methods of gradual withdrawal from ventilatory support during weaning from mechanical ventilation. Am J Respir Crit Care Med 1994;150:896

[59] Vogelsinger H, Kaehler CM. Hihg-flow oxygen therapy in COPD patients: Optimised oxygen delivery. European Respiratory Society Annual Congress 2013, Noninvasive Ventilatory Support, 386: 347

[60] Pisani L, Fasano L, Corcione N, et al. Change in pulmonary mechanics and the effect on breathing pattern of high flow oxygen therapy in stable hypercapnic COPD. Thorax 2017; 51: 373-375

[61] Longhini F, Pisani L, Lungu R, et al. High-flow oxygen therapy after noninvasive ventilation interruption in patients recovering from hypercapnic acute respiratory failure: A physiological Crossover trial. Crit Care Med 2019; 47: e506- e511

[62] Pisani L, Astuto M, Prediletto I, Longhini F. High flow through nasal cannula in exacerbated COPD patients: a systematic review. Pulmonol 2019;25(6):348-354

Chapter 8

Non-Pharmacological Management of Symptoms during Mechanical Ventilation and Chronic Obstructive Pulmonary Disease in Critical Care: Patient Directed Music Listening

Annie Heiderscheit

Abstract

This chapter provides a review of the literature on nonpharmacological management of symptoms with music listening for critically ill patients during mechanical ventilation and with chronic obstructive pulmonary disease. The critical care environment is high energy, intense, and noisy. These characteristics of the ICU can often exacerbate symptoms and overstimulate patients. Patients may experience increased agitation, anxiety, increased pain or discomfort, and sleep interruptions. Patients are often on various medications unique to their diagnosis and underlying health issues and may need additional medications to address symptoms associated with the hospitalization. Nonpharmacological management, such as music listening provides an intervention that can assist in managing multiple symptoms, can be utilized repeatedly or at various times through the day or evening, be tailored to patient preferences, can be safe and effective, and require minimal energy for patients to use. The chapter reviews the mechanisms of how music listening can help with symptom management and provides guidelines, recommendations, and contraindications for selecting music of patient use. A brief assessment tool is presented to help guide the process of determining patient music preferences and how music listening may be helpful. Lastly, recommendations are provided on how to make music listening accessible in the critical care environment.

Keywords: patient directed music listening, critical care, nonpharmacological, mechanical ventilation, COPD, symptom management

1. Introduction

Critical care is the highest level of care provided to the sickest of patients and thus requires and utilizes significant human and financial hospital resources, accounting for nearly 14% of overall hospital costs annually [1–3]. Patients with Chronic obstructive pulmonary disease (COPD) and those requiring mechanical ventilatory (MV) support are often admitted to intensive care units (ICU). It is estimated that COPD affects 400 million people around the world and by 2030, this number will surpass the annual global economic cost of cardiovascular disease, costing the world $50 trillion (USD) a year [4, 5]. Further, due to the progressive nature of COPD, severe exacerbation of symptoms often results in an ICU admission, which leads to 26–74% of patients requiring MV [6]. The complexity and severity of the disease led the World Health Organization (WHO) Burden of Disease Project to identify COPD as the fifth leading cause of death and projected that by 2020 it would be the third leading cause of death. ICU occupancy data indicates that between 20 and 39% of beds are filled with patients requiring mechanical ventilation [7].

In the United States alone, more than 1 million people are admitted to intensive care units each year and require MV [8]. Additionally, it is projected that by 2020 over 625,000 adults will required prolonged MV, which includes being ventilated for >96 hours [9]. The ICU environment is an active setting due to the acuity of patients and the need to ICU clinicians to provide constant and prompt care and attend to the changing needs of patients [10]. This critical care environment can be noisy due to the numerous medical devices on the unit and increased number of staff required to provide care [11, 12]. Critically ill patients experience a variety of symptoms that are due to their illness, sedative medications, and stress from noise associated with the ICU environment and that can hinder recovery [13–16]. As a result, critically ill patients experience a wide array of distressing symptoms throughout the course of their hospitalization, which include pain, discomfort, anxiety, stress, agitation, weakness, sleep deprivation, and delirium [17–19].

In recent years, clinicians and researchers have been making concerted efforts to recommend and utilize lighter levels of sedation to promote weaning ventilator support and overall recovery [20] and implementing non-pharmacological interventions such as music listening to manage symptoms associated with care on the ICU [21, 22]. The remainder of the chapter will focus on reviewing the literature regarding the use of music listening with critical ill patients, define patient directed music listening, provide guidelines for best practices in using music listening interventions, how to assess patient music preferences, considerations and contraindications for music listening, and review of economic benefits of music listening.

2. Use of music listening to manage symptoms

Music listening has emerged as a nonpharmacological approach to manage ICU acquired symptoms such as pain, agitation, anxiety, sleep disturbances, and confusion [23–25]. Due to the fact that these symptoms impact prolonged intensive care, length of hospitalization, morbidity, mortality, and the complexity of interactions with co-morbidities, it is challenging to manage this multiplicity of symptoms [26]. Music listening does not carry the side effects or negative consequences that first line interventions such as sedative and pain medications [25].

Music listening interventions have been implemented to manage a vast array of symptoms, and to manage multiple symptoms simultaneously to support the care and comfort for patients undergoing procedures, as well as those admitted to ICUs. Studies to date have evaluated the use of music listening to reduce discomfort and pain, stress and anxiety, the presence of delirium, sedative exposure, improve self-quality and cognitive functioning [27–42].

Author	Setting & subjects	Music intervention	Timing of music intervention	Outcomes
Singh V et al. [43]	72 COPD hospitalized patients randomized to a music or progressive muscle relaxation (PMR) group	Classical Indian music pre-selected by researchers	Patients listened to music for 30 minutes	• Significant decreased in both music and PMR groups, however changes were greater in music group on trait and state anxiety, dyspnea, SBP, PR and RR
Beaulieu-Borie et al. [44]	49 ICU patients randomized to music or control group (no music) from ICU	Slow tempo music pre-selected by researchers	Patients listened 1 hour 2 times per day	• Prolactin and blood cortisol decreased after intervention – Trend toward decreases in Fentanyl
Chlan et al. [28]	373 MV patients randomized to patient directed music listening (PDM), headphones (no music) or usual care group from 12 ICUs	Patient preferred music as assessed and tailored for patients by a board certified music therapist	Patients determined when and how long they wanted to listen to music	• PDM group had significantly lower anxiety scores • By 5th day anxiety decreased by 36.5% in PDM group • By 5th day PDM group had 2 fewer sedative doses
Han et al. [45]	137 ICU patients randomized to music listening, headphones, or control group	Relaxing music pre-selected by researchers	Patients listened for a single 30 minute session	• Significant decreases in HR, BP and RR over time in music group • Significant decrease in anxiety in music and headphone group • Significant increase in HR, BP, and RR in control group over time
Korhan et al. [46]	60 ICU patients randomized to music listening or control group	Classical music pre-selected by researchers	Patients listened to music for 60 minutes one time	• Patients in music group had significant decrease in RR and BP compared to control group
Lee et al. [47]	85 ICU MV patients randomized to music listening or control group	Relaxing music pre-selected by researchers	Patients listened to music 30 minutes one time per day	• Patients in the music group had demonstrated significantly reduced anxiety, serum cortisol, HR, and BP
Su et al. [48]	28 MICU patients randomized to music listening or control group	Four pieces of relaxing piano music	Patients listened to 45 minutes of music at nocturnal sleep time	• Patients in the music group had shorter N2 stage sleep and longer N3 stage sleep in the first two hours of sleep and improved self-reported sleep quality • Patients in the music group had significantly lower HR

Author	Setting & subjects	Music intervention	Timing of music intervention	Outcomes
Chlan et al. [49]	373 MV patients randomized to patient directed music listening (PDM), headphones (no music) or usual care group from 12 ICUs	Patient preferred music as assessed and tailored for patients by a board certified music therapist	Patients determined when and how long they wanted to listen to music	• PDM reduced anxiety by 19 points on VAS • PDM resulted in a cost savings of $2,322 (USD) per patient compared to usual care
Khan et al. [42]	117 ICU patients randomized to personalized music (PM), slow tempo music (STM) and attention control (AC) group		Listening sessions were 1 hour, 2 times a day for up to 7 days	• Adherence to study intervention was higher in PM and STM groups (80%) compared to AC group (30%) • Patients in the PM and STM groups had more coma free days than AC group

Table 1.
Review of music listening research.

Table 1 highlights recent research utilizing music listening interventions with critical care, COPD, and MV patients. The table includes details regarding the patient population, the music utilized in the music intervention, the timing of the music intervention and study outcomes. It is important to note the music utilized for the music intervention, the length and frequency of the music listening intervention varies significantly within this body of research.

Protocols regarding the selection of music vary in music listening intervention research. A Cochrane Review of music interventions with mechanically ventilated patients indicated that only 1 of the 14 studies reviewed included a board certified music therapist as a member of the research team [22]. As a result, in many studies the music was selected by the researchers and provided patients only limited options of music to listen to throughout the course of the study [50–53]. While researchers may refer to this as patient-preferred music, in essence patients are choosing what music to listen to, based on a pre-determined and a restrictive list of music, thus choosing what to listen to from limited options. Patient directed music listening is modeled after patient controlled analgesia (PCA), in which the patient makes their own decision regarding when they need to take a dose of pain medication [54]. Patient directed music listening (PDM) empowers the patient to choose the music they want to listen to, when they want to listen to it, and how long they want to listen [28, 54–56].

Implementing a music intervention with patients necessitates understanding the role or function of the music in the intervention. Additionally, implementing a patient directed music listening intervention requires understanding the patient's music preferences. This can be accomplished by completing a music assessment to help determine what the patient likes and does not like related to music listening. In order for a music intervention to be successful, it is vital to have a clear process of delivering the music intervention [21, 57]. These topics will be thoroughly explored in the upcoming sections of this chapter. The first step in this process is to understand how music listening can be helpful to patients in the ICU and the characteristics in music that support and facilitate these processes.

2.1 The role of music in a music listening intervention

Music is an accessible tool as critically ill patients can easily engage with music listening even when they are tired and have low energy [21, 54–57]. Music can serve many different functions to critically ill patients and can address multiple symptoms simultaneously [25]. Additionally, music does not hold the negative side effects or consequences that patients may experience from pharmacological interventions such as sedative and pain medications [25]. While a patient may use music listening to address multiple symptoms, it is important to understand the various roles music can play and characteristics in the music that can help address these symptoms [21, 49, 58–60]. **Table 2** identifies the different functions of music, descriptions, and characteristics in the music that facilitate this.

It is vital to understand the patient need(s) that music can help to address as this helps to determine music that may be most appropriate and effective for the patient. Conducting an assessment is critical to understanding a patient's needs and to determine their music preferences. A music assessment can also provide information on ways a patient may already use music in their day-to-day life, that can be helpful for them to use during their hospitalization.

There are several reasons why a music listening intervention is a viable option in the critical care environment. Listening to music can help enhance and promote a healing environment. As the patient is able to focus on the music and shift their focus

Function of music	Patient need addresses	Characteristics and considerations in the music
Relaxation: Relaxation response helps the body move from a stress response to a state of rest and calm.	Anxiety Stress Discomfort Pain Delirium	Slow rhythms in music foster a relaxation response by slowing the rhythms of the body as the breathing and heart rate entrain or synchronize with the slow rhythms in the music. This is an automatic response and the will body gradually synchronize with the slow rhythm it hears. Music that is 60–80 beats per minute (BPM) is ideal for fostering this relaxation response. Music that is preferred by the listener is more effective in fostering relaxation [21, 28, 49–52].
Distraction: Distraction is a helpful relaxation intervention as it focuses on shifting or directing attention or focus away from, or toward, something.	Anxiety Stress Discomfort Pain	Melody and lyrics are the elements in music that capture and hold our attention. Preferred instrumentation can also draw one's attention. Music that is preferred by the patient is most effective in diverting one's focus. It is important to select music that may not overstimulate given the ICU can be overstimulating [21, 49, 51].
Support sleep: Sleep is designed to be a restorative state in which the body rests and restores in preparation for each day.	Sleep deprivation Delirium Healing and recovery	The body and mind need to slow down and relax in order to move into a deep sleep state. Very slow rhythms (40–60 bpm) in music help to slow down the rhythms of the body to achieve a deep sleep state (delta sleep). Music that is consistent in dynamics and instrumentation further helps to lull the mind and body [21, 49].
Manage and shift mood: The state and quality of our feeling impact experiences. Negative mood states can intensify pain, discomfort, impede sleep, and impact healing.	Anxiety Stress Discomfort Pain	Tonality (major or minor), instrumentation and rhythm are the elements that connect to mood. One's familiarity to the music can impact a mood as well. Selecting music that represents (sounds like) the desired mood state can support shifting mood [53].

Table 2.
Functions of music.

away from the noisy or over stimulating environment of the ICU, this can foster a sense of relaxation and calm. Music can provide a sense of comfort as well. When a patient listens to soothing or familiar music, this can reduce stress and anxiety associated with their hospitalization. A music listening intervention provides the opportunity for the patient to exert control. Providing patients with the power to choose the music they want to listen to fosters feelings of empowerment, which is important when so many aspects of their care in the ICU is outside of their control [21, 55–58].

2.2 Assessing music preferences

Conducting an assessment is a key part of any treatment process. Implementing a music intervention is no exception. A music assessment allows the clinician to gather information that impacts a patient's music preferences, such as education, cultural background, and religious and faith affiliations. It provides insight into ways the patient may currently use music in their daily life that may be effective during the course of their treatment. The music assessment provides information on music preferences and music the patient does not like. Gathering this information helps to ensure the clinician can provide the music that can be more effective for the patient because it is their preferred music and to avoid music the patient does not like [21, 55, 58].

Music is often thought to be innocuous and does not have any negative impact. Listening to music one does not like can cause agitation and negatively impact mood [21, 55]. Music can also be connected to significant life experiences and hearing songs that remind a patient of those experiences can foster a strong emotional response. As a result, it is important to understand which music may not be appropriate or helpful for the patient [55, 57].

The Brief Music Assessment Tool (BMAT) that follows can be utilized to effectively and efficiently assess a patient's music preferences. The BMAT is an abbreviated version of a music assessment tool (MAT) utilized in patient directed music listening research [28, 55, 57]. Recent research indicates that patients did not find the gathering of assessment data burdensome, as it could be collected quickly and easily [25] (**Table 3**).

Patient demographic information
Patient name: Date: Education: Vocation: Cultural background: Religion or faith background: Current mood state: Hearing impairment: Specify:
Music preferences assessment
1. Do you like to listen to music? Yes No
2. Do you play an instrument(s)? Yes No If yes, what do you play?
3. When do you like to listen to music? (Check all that apply) ____Relaxation ___ Stress reduction ____ Pure enjoyment ____ To pass time ____ During exercise ____ During meals ____ With friends & family ____ For prayer ____ While working ____ Other (please specify) ______________________________ ______________________________

4. What types of music do you enjoy? (Check all that apply)

____ Classical	____ Religious/Sacred
____ Classic rock	____ Hard rock
____ Rhythm & blues	____ Country
____ Hip hop	____ Reggae
____ Jazz	____ Rap
____ New age	____ World music
____ Alternative	____ Heavy metal
____ Oldies (1950–1970)	____ Pop music
____ Other (please specify)	

____

____

5. Are there any particular groups or artists you prefer?

____

____

6. What instruments or instrumental sounds do you like? (Check all that apply)

____ Orchestral	____ Harp
____ Vocal	____ Flute
____ Folk/acoustic guitar	____ Piano
____ Synthesizer	____ Strings (violin, viola, cello)
____ Electric guitar	____ Bass
____ Saxophone	____ Percussion/drumming
____ Brass or horns	____ Clarinet or oboe
____ Ocean waves	____ Environmental sounds
____ Others (please specify)	

____

____

7. Are there any instruments or instrumental sounds that you DO NOT like? (Please specify)

____

____

8. Are there any genres of music you DO NOT like? (Please specify)

____

____

9. Are there any groups or artists you DO NOT like? (Please specify)

____

____

10. Are there any cultural considerations important for you when selecting music? (Please specify)

____

____

Table 3.
Brief music assessment tool (BMAT).

When the music assessment is complete and the clinician has a clear understanding of what patient needs that music can help to address, as well as what music the patient prefers and will be most effective, the next step is determining the delivery method of the music listening intervention. The method of delivery should be accessible at all times to enable the patient to utilize music listening when they want or need, and for their desired length of time [21, 56, 58].

2.3 Considerations of delivery of a music listening intervention

Music is easily accessible through many different platforms and various devices. Patients may have their preferred music available on their personal mobile devices (iPhone, Smartphone, iPad, laptop, etc.) which they have available during their hospitalization. If so, it can be helpful to talk with the patient about the music they have available and how they can use it to manage symptoms. An intensive care unit may choose to make music available through a platform or device on the unit. There are several considerations when making music available for patient use.

It is imperative that the delivery process be accessible to patients whenever they may want or need to engage in music listening. Accessibility is a vital consideration when creating a delivery system, as well as one that does not burden ICU staff. Patients need to be able to access the music and any equipment needed to engage in music listening with as little assistance as possible. This will empower them to use the music listening for their own care, if they are not dependent upon family or staff to help them access it. It is important to provide music that is tailored to patients' music preferences. This can require having a diverse and extensive collection of music or access to music streaming. Providing limited genres of music for patients does not allow them to select their preferred music and can discourage use of the intervention. Additionally, given the noisy nature of the ICU it can be helpful for patients to use headphones or ear buds when listening to music. These devices can help block out environmental noise and to further enhance the listening experience, as well as to help avoid over stimulation [21, 56, 58]. **Table 4** provides more detailed information and considerations for the music listening delivery process.

Delivery process	Considerations	Suggestions
Music source **Streaming** (Spotify, Apple music, etc.) Playlists on iPad **Patient's own**	**Broad selection** Music selection needs to include a wide array of music to accommodate patients' preferred music **Management** If a collection is maintained by the institution, staff may be needed to manage and update **Budget** Music provided by the institution will require funding to purchase music or streaming service and equipment. Patients may have their own device and music for use.	Costs of streaming services available for institutional use should be reviewed and any restrictions that may apply. Institutions should evaluate what options are feasible and affordable based on patient care needs to determine the most viable option. Be sure to review copyright laws if purchasing music to be loaded onto iPads and make available for patient use.
Equipment: **Music storage** Internal platform (i.e. GetWell Network iPad **Patient's own** Patients or families may have a mobile device with preferred music **Headphones** Headphones and ear buds help to block out environmental noise and can enhance the music listening experience, allowing the patient to focus on the music	**Music platform** The platform selected needs to be easy for patients to use and manage, as they are often tired and have low energy **Individual availability** Many patients have their own mobile device, music and headphones/ear buds that they choose to use in lieu of institutional equipment. **Accessibility** The equipment and platform needs to be accessible to the patient to ensure they can engage in music listening when they want and need. **Security** Equipment that is provided by the institution needs to be secured so it is available to patient and so it is not misplaced, lost, or stolen.	Skills of patients to manage and operate the equipment must be considered when choosing the music delivery process. Patients may prefer to use their own equipment as it is familiar and includes their preferred music. Patient's may need some instruction on how to operate the equipment [25]. It can be helpful to provide written instructions for operating music listening equipment for patients and families to refer to. This can empower them in accessing and using the music. Equipment that is provided needs to follow institutional guidelines for infection and disease control. As a result consideration should be given to the ability to properly clean and disinfect equipment.

Delivery process	Considerations	Suggestions
Information and education: **Patients** Patients may have some idea of how music listening can be helpful but will benefit from additional information to be able to use it effectively. They may also feel overwhelmed, tired, confused, and as a result can benefit from information and reminders of how music listening can be helpful. **Staff** Care staff may or may not have a clear understanding of the benefits of music listening or how the music listening process has been set up for patient use on the unit. It is important to inform and educate staff to enable them to integrate music listening into their patient care regime.	**Educating patients** Most people listen to music and understand it is an enjoyable and relaxing. It is helpful to provide patients some simple information and education to help them understand the many different ways that listening to music can manage symptoms. This information and knowledge will encourage their use of music listening and empower them in their own care. **Staff** Staff can benefit from some education and training to ensure they are able to properly educate and inform patients regarding the use of music listening. It also empowers staff to know when it may be appropriate to suggest or recommend a patient try music listening [61].	Literature is available to help inform staff about implementing a patient directed music listening intervention [21, 25, 55, 56]. Institutions and critical care units may choose to consult a board certified music therapist (MT-BC) to utilize their expertise about the use of music and music listening with patients. Organizations can contact state or local music therapy organizations or contact the American Music Therapy Association to get assistance in locating a music therapist in the area.

Table 4.
Delivery process for patient directed music listening.

There are additional considerations for patients that are sedated during MV and are unable to complete the music assessment or make decisions regarding music preferences or when to listen to music. In these situations, staff should inquire with family or caregivers to ascertain as much of the information possible for the music assessment. While patients that are sedated are not able to communicate their desire to listen to music, if the staff are observing signs that patient is anxious, stressed, experiencing pain and discomfort, this is an opportunity to explore the use of music listening. Staff assist in providing the music for patients by ensuring it is the patient's preferred music and the volume level of the music is appropriate for the patient. Staff should take a few moments to observe the patient listening to notice how the patient may be responding to the music and confirm it is the appropriate intervention at this time. Music via headphones or in the patient room should not be played for hours on end for sedated patients. Music listening is an intervention that a sedated patient does not have control over, and is therefore dependent on staff and family members and loved ones to properly attend to the delivery.

These various considerations, and the choices a unit or institution makes surrounding them, will be unique to the patients, the staff, the ICU unit, and the organization. Therefore, it is important to determine the resources available to dedicate to a music listening intervention and to ensure that unit staff are invested, dedicated, and educated in how it can benefit patients as well as how to implement the intervention with patients [21, 25, 56].

3. Conclusion

While the costs of the complex care of patients with COPD and who are mechanically ventilated continue to rise, these costs account significant portions of hospital budgets [1, 2]. As a result, viable options are needed that can enhance patient care, that do not impose further complications or negative consequences, and are cost-effective. Music listening has emerged as an ideal intervention as it meets this criteria. Music listening has garnered significant interest as a non-pharmacological intervention for critically ill patients due to its ease of delivery, limited cost of delivery, the variety of symptoms it helps to address, the potential to reduce sedation, and to reduce overall cost of ICU care [21, 55–60, 62]. Additionally, patients and their families report that music listening helps to reduce anxiety and improve sleep, and they appreciated being given the opportunity to choose music as a part of their treatment and care [25, 61, 62].

While music listening is an optimal intervention for critically ill patients, patient directed music listening, allows the patient to choose their preferred music and engage in listening to music whenever, and for as long as they want. This approach to music listening empowers patients in their care process and has demonstrated significant outcomes as a result of its tailored approach [28, 58, 61, 63]. It is important for the healthcare organization and ICU staff to understand how to implement a patient directed music listening intervention and carefully determine the best method of delivery for their respective setting.

Acknowledgements

The author would like to acknowledge the colleagues she has collaborated with on various research studies, which contributed considerably to the body of literature regarding the use of music listening with mechanically ventilated and critically ill patients. Dr. Linda Chlan (Mayo Clinic), principal investigator on Award Number R01 NR009295 supported by National Institute of Nursing Research of the National Institutes of Health with Dr. Debra Skaar, Dr. Craig Weinert and Dr. Mary Fran Tracy. Dr. Babar Khan (Indiana University Medical School), principal investigator on Award Number R01AG067631 supported by the National Institute on Aging and Eye Institute along with Dr. Sikandar Khan and Dr. Linda Chlan.

Funding

Funding provided by Annie Heiderscheit, Ph.D., MT-BC, LMFT and Augsburg University.

Conflict of interest

The author declares no conflict of interest.

Author details

Annie Heiderscheit
Augsburg University, Minneapolis, MN, United States

*Address all correspondence to: heidersc@augsburg.edu

References

[1] Pastores S, Dakwa J, Halpern H. Costs of Critical Care Medicine. *Critical Care Clinics.* 2012; 28(1): 1-10. doi: 10.1016/j.ccc.2011.10.003.

[2] Cerro G, Checkely, M. Global analysis of critical care burden. *Lancet Respir Med.* 2014; 2(5): 343-344. doi:10.1016/S2213-2600(14)70042-6

[3] Marshall J, Bosco L, Adhikari N, Bronwen C, Diaz J, Dorman T, Fowler R, Geert, M, Nakagawa S, Pelosi P, Vincent J, Vollman K, Zimmerman J. What is an intensive care unit? A report of the task force of the World Federation of Societies of Intensive and Critical Care Medicine. *Journal of Crit Care Med,* 2017; 37: 270-276. doi: 10.1016/j.jcrc.2016.07.015

[4] Bloom D, Cafiero E, Jané-Llopis E, Abrahams-Gessel S, Bloom L, Fathima S, Feigel A, Gaziano T, Mowafi M, Pandya A, Prettner K, Rosenberg L, Seligman B, Stein A, Weinstein C. The global economic burden of non-communicable diseases. 2011. *World economic forum.*

[5] Barnes P. COPD 2020: New directions needed. *Am J Physical Lung Cell Mol Physiol*. 2020; 319: L884-L886. DOI: 101152/ajplung.00473.2020.

[6] Othman F, Ismaiel Y, Alkhathran S, Alshamrani A, Alghamdi M, Ismaiel T. The duration of mechanical ventilation in patients with chronic obstructive pulmonary disease and acute respiratory distress syndrome admitted to the intensive care unit: Epidemiological findings from a tertiary hospital. *J Nat Sc Biol Med.* 2020;11:61-65. DOI: 10.4103/jnsbm.JNSBM_199_19.

[7] Wunsch H, Wagner J, Herlim M, Chong D, Kramer A, Halpern S. ICU occupancy and mechanical ventilator use in the United States. *Crit Care Med.* 2013: 41(12). doi: 10.1097/CCM.0b013e318298a139.

[8] Cox C, Carson S, Govert J, Chelluri L, Sanders G. An economic evaluation of prolonged mechanical ventilation. *Crit Care Med*. 2007; 35(8): 1918-1927.

[9] Zilberg M, de Witt M, Shorr A. Accuracy of previous estimates for adult prolonged acute mechanical ventilation volume in 2020: Update using 200-2008 data. *Crit Care Med.* 2012; 40(1): 18-20.

[10] Burk R, Grap, M, Munro C, et al. Agitation onset, frequency, and associated temporal factors in critically ill adults. *Am J Crit Care.* 2014; 23: 296-304.

[11] Busch-Visniac, I, West J, Barnhill C, et al. Noise levels in Johns Hopkins Hospital. *J Acoust Soc Am.* 2005;118: 3629-3645.

[12] Konkani A, Oakley B. Noise in hospital intensive care units – a critical review of a critical topic. *J Crit Care.* 2012; 27:522e1-522e9.

[13] Berglund B, Lindvall T, Schwela D. Guidelines for community noise. Paper presented at: World Health Organization Expert Task Force meeting: April 26-30, 1999, London, United Kingdom.

[14] Choiniere D. The effects of hospital noise. *Nurse Admin Q.* 2010; 34; 327-333.

[15] Morrison W, Haas E, Shaffner D, et al. Noise, stress, and annoyance in pediatric intensive care unit. *Crit Care Med.* 2003; 31:113-119.

[16] Novelo J. High frequency oscillatory ventilation (HFOV) generates potentially harmful noise in the medical intensive care unit. *Chest.* 2012; 142(4 meeting abstracts):949A

[17] Lopez A, Shibuya K, Rao C, et al. Chronic obstructive pulmonary disease: current burden and future projections. *Eur Respir J. 2006;* 27: 397-412.

[18] Lopez A, Mathers C, Ezzati M, Jamison D, Murray C. Global burden of disease and risk factors. *The World Bank.* 2006.

[19] Buist A, McBurnie M, Vollmer W, Gillespie S, Burney P, Mannino D, Menezes A, Sullivan S, Lee T, Weiss R, Marks G, Gulsvik A, Nizankowska-Mogilnicka W. International variation in the prevalence of COPD (The BOLD Study): a population-based prevalence study. *The Lancet.* 2007; 370; 741-750. doi: 10.1016/S0140-6736(07)61377-4.

[20] Barr J, Fraser G, Puntillo K, et al. American College of Critical Care Medicine: Clinical practice guidelines for management of pain, agitation, and delirium in adult patients in the intensive care unit. *Crit Care Med.* 2013; 41: 392-398.

[21] Chlan L, Tracy M, Heiderscheit A, Hetland B. Nonpharmacological interventions for pain, agitation, and delirium. In: Balas M, Clemmer T, Hargett K, editors. *ICU Liberation: The power of pain control, minimal sedation, and early mobility.* Society of Critical Care Medicine; 2017. p. 161-166.

[22] Bradt J, Dileo C. Music interventions for mechanically ventilated patients. *Cochrane Database of Systematic Reviews* 2014; 12. doi: 10.1002/14651858.CD006902.pub3.

[23] Chanques G, Jaber S, Barbotte E, et al. Impact of systematic evaluation of pain and agitation in an intensive care unit. *Crit Care Med.* 2006; 34(6): 1691-1699. doi: 10.1097/01.CCM.0000218416.62457.56.

[24] Kamdar B, Needham D, Collop N. Sleep deprivation in critical illness: its role in physical and physiological recovery. *J Intensive Care Med.* 2012; 27(2):97-111.

[25] Knudson K, Redeker N, Heiderscheit A, Pisani M, Knauert M, Chlan L. Acceptability and feasibility of a patient-directed music intervention in the medical intensive care unit (manuscript in review).

[26] Reade M, Finfer S. Sedation and delirium in the intensive care unit. *NEJM.* 2014; 370(5):444-454. doi: 10.1056?NEJMra1208705.

[27] Chiasson A, Baldwin A, McLaughlin C, Cook P, Sethi G. The effect of live spontaneous harp music on patients in the intensive care unit. *Evid-Based Compl Alt.* 2013. Article ID 428731. doi: 10.1155/2023/428731.

[28] Chlan L, Weinert C, Heiderscheit A, et al. Effects of patient-directed music intervention on anxiety and sedative exposure in critically ill patients receiving mechanical ventilatory support: a randomized clinical trial. *JAMA.* 2013; 309(22):2335-2344. doi: 10.1001/jama.2013.5670.

[29] Golino A, Leone R, Gollenberg A, et al. Impact of an active music therapy intervention on intensive care patients. *Am J Crit Care.* 2019;28(1):48-55. doi: 10.4037/ajcc2019792.

[30] Hu R, Jiang X, Hegadoren K, Zhang Y. Effects of earplugs and eye masks combined with relaxing music on sleep, melatonin and cortisol levels in ICU patients: a randomized controlled trial. *Crit Care.* 2015;19:115. doi: 10.1186/s13054-015-0855-3.

[31] McCaffery R. The effect of music on acute confusion in older adults after hip or knee surgery. *Appl Nurs Res.* 2009; 22(2): 107-112. doi. 10.1016/j.apnr.2007.06.004.

[32] Nilsson U. The anxiety and pain reducing effects of music interventions: a systematic review. *AORN J.* 2008;87(4):780-807. Doi.10.1016/j.oarn.2007.09.013.

[33] Ozer N, Karaman O, Arslan S. Günes N. Effect of music on postoperative pain and physiologic parameters of patients after open heart surgery. *Pain Manag Nurs.* 2013;14(1):20-28. doi: 10.1016/jpmn.2010.05.002.

[34] Ryu M, Park J, Park H. Effect of sleep-inducing music on sleep in persons with percutaneous transluminal coronary angiography in cardiac care unit. *J Clin Nurs.* 2012;21(5-6);728-735. DOI: 10.1111/j.1365-2702.2011.03876.x.

[35] Sendelback S, Halm M, Doran K, Miller E, Gaillard, P. Effects of music therapy on physiological and psychological outcomes for patients undergoing cardiac surgery. *J Cardiovasc Nurs.* 2006; 21(3): 194-200. doi: 10.1097/00005082-200605000-00007.

[36] Su C, Lai H, Chang E, Yin L, Perng S, Chen P. A randomized controlled trial of the effects of listening to non-commercial music on quality of nocturnal sleep and relaxation indices in patients in medical intensive care unit. *J Adv Nurs.* 2013;69(6):1377-1389. Doi: 10.1111/j.1365-2648.2012.06130.x.

[37] Tan X, Yowler C, Super D, Fratianne R. The efficacy of music therapy protocols for decreasing pain, anxiety, and muscle tension levels during burn dressing changes: a prospective randomized crossover trial. *J Burn Care Res.* 2010;31(4):590-597. DOI: 10.1016/jpmn.2010.05.002.

[38] Twiss E, Seaver J, McCaffrey R. The effect of music listening on older adults undergoing cardiovascular surgery. *Nurs Crit Care.* 2006;11(5):224-231. Doi: 10.111/j.1478-5153.2006.00174.x.

[39] Vaajoki A, Pietilä A, Vehiläinen-Julkunen K. Effects of listening to music on pain intensity and pain distress after surgery: an intervention. *J Clin Nurs.* 2012;21(5-6):708-717. Doi: 10.1111/j.1365-2702.2011.03829.x.

[40] Kamioka H, Tsutani K, Yamadan M. et al. Effectiveness of music therapy: a summary of systematic reviews based on randomized controlled trials of music interventions. *Patient Prefer Adherence.* 2014: 8:727-754. Doi: 10.2147/PPA. S61340.

[41] Khan S, Wang S, Harrawood A, Martinez S, Heiderscheit A, Chlan L, Perkins A, Tu W, Boustani M, Khan B. Decreasing delirium through music (DDM) in critically ill, mechanically ventilated patients in the intensive care unit: protocol for a randomized controlled trial. *Clinical Trials.* 2017; 18(574), 2-8.

[42] Khan S, Durrai S, Xu C, Purpura R, Lindroth H, Wang S, Perkins A, Goa S, Heiderscheit A, Chlan L, Boustani M, Khan B. Decreasing delirium through music (DDM): a randomized controlled pilot trial. *Amer J of Crit Care.* 2020; 29(2);31-39.

[43] Singh V, Rao V, Prem V, Sahoo R, Pai K K. Comparison of the effectiveness of music and progressive muscle relaxation for anxiety in COPD – A randomized controlled pilot study. *Chr Res Dis.* 2009;6(4):209-216

[44] Beaulieu-Boire G, Bourgue S, Chagnon F, Chouinard L, Gallo-Payet N, Lesur O. Music and biological stress dampening in mechanically ventilated patients at intensive care unit ward – a prospective interventional randomized crossover trial. *J Crit Care.* 2013;28(4):442-450.

[45] Han L, Li, J, Sit J, Chung L, Jiao Z, Ma W. Effectives of music intervention on physiological stress response and anxiety level of mechanically ventilated patients in China: a randomized controlled trial. *J Clin Nurs.* 2010; 19(7-8): 978-987.

[46] Korhan E, Khorshid L, Uyar M. The effect of music therapy on physiological signs of anxiety in patients receiving mechanical ventilatory support. *J Clin Nurs.* 2011;20(7-8):1026-1034.

[47] Lee H, Lee C, Hsu M, Lai C, Sung Y, Lin C, Lin L. Effects of music intervention on state anxiety and physiological indices in patients undergoing mechanical ventilation in intensive care unit: a randomized controlled trial. *Bio Res Nurs.* 2017;19(2):137-144.

[48] Su C, Lai H, Chang E, Yiin L, Perng S, Chen P. A randomized controlled trial of the effects of listening to non-commercial music on quality of nocturnal sleep and relaxation indices in patients in medical intensive care unit. *J Adv Nurs.* 2012; 69(6):1377-1389.

[49] Chlan L, Heiderscheit A, Skaar D, Neidecker M. Economic evaluation of patient directed music intervention compared to usual care costs in ICU patients receiving mechanical ventilatory support. *Crit Care Med.* 2018;46(9):1430-1435. Doi: 10.1097/ccm.0000000000003199

[50] Jafari H, Zeydi A, Khani S, et al. The effects of listening to preferred music on pain intensity after open heart surgery. *Nurs Midw Res.* 2012;17(1),1-6.

[51] Khan S, Kitsis M, Golovyan D, et al. Effects of music intervention on inflammatory markers of critically ill and post-operative patients: a systematic review of the literature. *Heart Lung.* 2018;47(5):489-496.

[52] Nilsson U. The anxiety and pain reducing effects of music interventions: a systematic review. *AORN.* 2008:87(4):780-807.

[53] Kühlmann A, de Rooij A, Kroese L, et al. Meta-analysis evaluation of music interventions for anxiety and pain in surgery. *Br J Surg.* 2018;105:773-783.

[54] Heiderscheit A, Chlan L, Donley K. Instituting a music listening intervention for critically ill patients receiving mechanical ventilation: Exemplars from two patient cases. *Mus Med.* 2011;3(4):239 245.

[55] Chlan L, Heiderscheit A. A tool for music preference assessment in critically ill patients receiving mechanical ventilatory support: an interdisciplinary approach. *Mus Ther Persp.* 2009;27(1):42-47.

[56] Chlan L, Heiderscheit A. Music intervention. In Lindquist R, Snyder M, Tracy M, editors. *Complementary & Alternative Therapies in Nursing.* 8th ed. New York: Springer. 2018. P. 109-126.

[57] Heiderscheit A, Brechenridge S, Chlan L, Savik K. Music preferences of mechanically ventilated patients participating in a randomized controlled trial. *Mus Med.* 2014;6(2):29-38.

[58] Heiderscheit A. Music therapy in surgical and procedural support for adult medical patients. In Allen J, editor. *Guidelines for music therapy with adult medical patients.* Gilsum: Barcelona; 2013. P. 17-34.

[59] Heiderscheit A, Jackson N. *Introduction to Music Therapy Practice.* Barcelona; 2018. P. 305.

[60] Heiderscheit A, Madson A. Use of the iso principle as a central method of mood management: a music psychotherapy clinical case study. *Mus Ther Persp.* 2015;33(1):45-52.

[61] Tracy M, Staugitis A, Chlan L, Heiderscheit A. Perceptions of patients and families who received a music intervention during mechanical ventilation. *Mus Med.* 2015;7(3):54-58.

[62] Kahn, J, et al. Cost savings attributable to reductions in intensive care unit length of stay for mechanically ventilated patients. *Med Care.* 2008; 46(2):1226-1233

[63] Meghani N, Tracy M, O'Connor-Von S, Niakosari N, Mathiason M, Lindquist R. Generating evidence of critical care nurses' perceptions, knowledge, beliefs, and use of music therapy, aromatherapy, and guided imagery. *Dim Crit Care Nurs.* 2020; (Jan/Feb):47-57. doi: 10.1097/01. Dcc.0000615856.49651.9f.